The Management of ADHD in Children and Young People

The Management of ADHD in Children and Young People

Edited by Val Harpin

2017
Mac Keith Press

© 2017 Mac Keith Press

Managing Director: Ann-Marie Halligan
Production Manager/Commissioning Editor: Udoka Ohuonu
Project Management: Riverside Publishing Solutions Ltd

First published in this edition in 2016 by Mac Keith Press
6 Market Road, London, N7 9PW

British Library Cataloguing-in-Publication data
A catalogue record for this book is available from the British Library

Cover design: Hannah Rogers

ISBN: 978-1-909962-72-9

Typeset by Riverside Publishing Solutions Ltd

Printed by Hobbs the Printers Ltd, Totton, Hampshire, UK
Mac Keith Press is supported by Scope.

Contents

Contents

Author Appointments

Caroline Bleakley
Associate Specialist in Paediatric Neurodisability, Ryegate Children's Centre, Sheffield, UK

Helen Crimlisk
Consultant, General Adult Psychiatry, Sheffield Health and Social Care Foundation NHS Trust, Sheffield, UK

David Daley
Professor of Psychological Intervention and Behaviour Change, Division of Psychiatry and Applied Psychology, School of Medicine, University of Nottingham; Co-director, Centre for ADHD and Neurodevelopmental Disorders, Institute of Mental Health, University of Nottingham, UK

Val Harpin
Consultant Neurodevelopmental Paediatrician, Ryegate Children's Centre, Sheffield, UK

Peter Hill
Consultant Child and Adolescent Psychiatrist, 127 Harley Street, London, UK

KAH Mirza
Consultant Psychiatrist, Department of Child Psychiatry, Hertfordshire Partnership University NHS Trust, Hertfordshire; Honorary Senior Lecturer, Institute of Psychiatry, King's College London, UK

Sudeshni Mirza
Professor of Forensic Medicine, DM Wayanad Institute of Medical Sciences, Naseera Nagar, Kerlala, India

Nikos Myttas
Consultant Child and Adolescent Psychiatrist, 127 Harley Street, London, UK

Fintan O'Regan
Learning and Behaviour Trainer and Consultant; former Head Teacher of the Centre Academy School, London, UK

Eric Rosenthal
Consultant Paediatric & Adult Congenital Cardiologist, Evelina London Children's Hospital, St Thomas' Hospital, London, UK

Mel Seymour
ADHD Nurse Specialist, Sheffield Children's NHS Foundation Trust, UK

Shatha Shibib
Consultant Child and Adolescent Psychiatrist, Sheffield Children's NHS Foundation Trust, UK

Roshin M. Sudesh
Speciality Trainee in Emergency Medicine, Medway Maritime Hospital, Gillingham, UK

Julie Warburton
ADHD Nurse Specialist, Sheffield Children's NHS Foundation Trust, UK

Foreword

As a training psychiatrist in the early 1990s, then as a Consultant child and adolescent psychiatrist and finally a Clinical Director in a Child and Adolescent Mental Health Service, I have seen how the recognition, diagnosis and treatment of ADHD has been changing the shape of child mental health and paediatric services over the last 20 years. It has challenged clinicians' understanding of behavioural difficulties and their perception of neurodevelopmental disorders. It has required education services to rethink how they manage children and young people with ADHD who are struggling in school.

ADHD is a disorder surrounded in controversy and debate, in both the clinical setting and the wider community. Medicines are viewed as transforming by some, but as chemical restraint by others. Despite extensive research into the condition the world appears to be no closer to an agreement on the nature of the disorder and how best to treat it. While the arguments persist the children, young people and, more recently, adults continue to seek help for the problems that develop from the disorder, such as remaining focused or regulating their behavior.

There is a wide range of books associated with the science or clinical management of ADHD. Some are purely neuroscience and focus on the current state of knowledge. But in this field the science is moving on so rapidly that by the time of publication these books are always slightly behind the cutting-edge research in on the subject. Others are self-help books for assisting families or individuals who are affected by the condition.

The *Management of ADHD in Children and Young People* is written by clinicians and for clinicians and as a consequence it reflects the knowledge and needs of those providing care for those with ADHD. The authors have taken a practical approach to the disorder. They have not only referenced the most up-to-date literature but have also used their extensive clinical experience to describe what ADHD is, how to recognise it, what to do when you see it, and how to treat it and its coexisting difficulties. They give insights into the history of the condition and then using the UK as an example they have built a profile of how ADHD presents in the modern world and the challenges it now presents to clinicians.

'Every child with ADHD is different' is a phrase used by clinicians to reassure parents that the understanding of their child and the treatment offered is being tailored to their individual needs. Although this is true, there is much that can be learnt from clinical examples that highlight the frequently occurring problems associated with the condition and its treatment. This is reflected in this volume. The authors' use of clinical vignettes throughout the chapters brings a reality to the condition that makes the book relevant to clinicians working with individuals with ADHD. It provides practical suggestions on how to approach the condition or how to develop services to meet the needs of the ever increasing number of people seeking help.

The topics covered in this book reflect the questions clinicians working in the specialities of child and adolescent psychiatry or paediatrics frequently want answered and so would be ideal for training grade clinicians. The authors have used their experience of delivering teaching to ensure that their content is clear and understandable to all. This book is not a simple introduction to the subject; clinicians from all backgrounds in children's services, and at all levels of seniority will find something of value or interest, whether it be seeking validation for their current clinical practice or new insights into how to approach clinical challenges. As the science basis expands, our understanding of the neurobiology of this condition will increase; however, the need for access to the experience of clinicians who have been delivering care to this group of children and young people will remain irreplaceable. This book thoroughly fulfills that need.

Dr Duncan Manders
Consultant Child and Adolescent Psychiatrist
Royal Hospital for Sick Children
Edinburgh, UK

Preface

I didn't choose ADHD. It chose me. I am so pleased it did.

I started to work with children and young people with ADHD and their families in the early 1990's, just as awareness was increasing in the UK and the rest of Europe. We had little to offer at that time: some behavioural management and short acting methylphenidate as the only available medication, but at least ADHD was being recognised.

So much has changed in the last 25 years. In that time, we have all realised how complex ADHD is and how important thorough assessment and optimal treatment is to improved outcomes. We also have many more treatment options.

My fascination for the topic has grown and grown and I have been fortunate to learn so much from the children, young people and their families and from teachers and colleagues.

The aim of this book is to share sound, practical management advice built on a strong evidence base and many years of practical experience. The management of ADHD needs input from a strong multidisciplinary team to offer children and young people and their families the services they need.

Our book starts with the viewpoint of David Tompkinson, a young man who has grown up with ADHD. He describes some of his experiences and how he now celebrates his ADHD and succeeds. I am very grateful to David for sharing this with us.

The chapter authors come from a variety of multidisciplinary backgrounds, with contributions from paediatrics, child and adolescent psychiatry, psychology, specialist nursing, teaching and adult psychiatry, each sharing their expertise and advice on a particular aspect of ADHD management. The result is a comprehensive overview of issues we face as clinicians involved in the management of ADHD and its many comorbid conditions.

Although the services described are based on UK school and health systems, the principles involved and the practical management advice offered are international: ADHD is universal.

I would like to thank all of the authors for their excellent input, for freely giving their valuable time and for their ongoing support throughout the process.

My thanks also to the team at Mac Keith, especially Udoka Ohuonu, who has been throughout a calm and positive guide and to Lisa Trueman for patience and thoroughness as the book became 'real'.

Thank you, of course, to all the children, young people and families I have had the pleasure of working with at the Ryegate Centre in Sheffield and to the fantastic staff Team I have been privileged to work with over the years.

Lastly, special thanks to my wonderful family, Martin, Briony, Nick and Krystina.

Val Harpin
September 2016

Prologue: ADHD and proud

When Doctor Harpin asked me to write this piece for this very important and much needed book, I jumped at the chance. Of course I did. Without thinking. No hesitation. I said yes. That's what life with ADHD is like. But whilst so much of ADHD is given a bad reputation, I'm here to let you into a little secret: it can be used to a person's advantage.

I can 100% say, even when I stop for a moment and think (a rare occasion indeed), that I am so proud to have ADHD. Of course it can be a struggle, and my journey with ADHD has had an abundance of them. But with the right help and the right support it can be channelled into success.

Before I digress further, and please do bare with me if I do this, I don't always mean to it's just that….. whoops. There I go again.

Allow me to introduce myself, my name is David Tompkinson, and I have ADHD. I want to tell what I think is a very positive story about a condition that I have struggled with, wrestled with, grown up with and eventually tamed.

I came to Dr Harpin when I was a 6-year-old. I was not fascinated with the lady who has now come very close to my heart, but instead with the Mr Potato toy in her office. (I never had the heart to tell her I once 'liberated' his left shoe).

I was referred to Dr Harpin because essentially I was a problem; a problem for my parents, teachers, brother and pretty much anyone who I was with for a long period of time. I couldn't sit still. I was very hyperactive. I was impulsive. I was so ADHD.

At the time (and do note when I say, at the time) this was a problem because I was trouble at school and simply didn't engage with any of my learning or teachers. But also, school didn't engage with me. I was labelled a 'hopeless' case and a drain on the teachers' time and efforts.

In Infant school and Junior school, I was outside of the class more times than I was in it. Thankfully, the days of making children wait in corridors has long gone.

My parents used to have countless messages from my school on the answer phone when they got home; 'David's done this, David's done that.' My father being the diligent organiser he is (a trait I never picked up), kept all the letters and exchanges between the schools and reading them back now, I can see it was just a constant battle for them. I once shed a tear reading the ending to one of my Dad's letters to school which read: 'Whatever people think about our son, he is incredibly special to us and we will always look to see the beauty in a boy that my wife and I love endlessly'.

My parents have been my rock throughout my journey with ADHD and have kept me on the straight path so many times. Without their support I wouldn't be where I am today. That's my first massive avocation, supportive parents. At times it must have been so hard for my parents to put on a brave face, but they believed in me and never lost hope. Unconditional love as my Mother always puts it.

As I grew older I started to manage the condition a little better. I discovered a love of history, politics, thought and debate- much to my brother's annoyance. But he was, and still, is an incredibly intelligent man. I started to engage with him and talk to him about all the things I was interested in. He developed my love of learning and ignited passions for things I never really thought I could bring to the surface.

GCSE's were a battle and a struggle. I had lost so much of my early years in learning, and the foundations were not there. Especially in mathematics and getting a C in maths is up there with my greatest achievements, gaining me entry to Sixth form where I could study the subjects I loved. Was University in sight for a boy who was deemed a failure and a 'no hoper'?

June 6th 2012 was one of the happiest days of my life. I sat stunned, looking at a computer screen that was telling me I had been accepted at the University of Durham. My Mother was in floods of tears, unable to speak for pride. That was their day; 21 years of sleepless nights, worry, phone calls, backhanded comments from other parents. That was their moment.

On the day I graduated I handed Dad my robes to try on, and I said: 'I wouldn't be here today if it wasn't for you Dad.'

I am currently training to be a primary school teacher (ironic huh?) having just graduated from Durham University with a First Class Honours degree. This is the boy who couldn't sit still (and still can't really) for longer than 30 seconds. This is the boy who was told by a teacher he 'would go nowhere in life' because he's 'stupid'.

Life with ADHD is truly a rollercoaster. I still can't sit still. I still can't really concentrate. But I have found a way to make life work for me.

There is hope. Just believe in the ADHD child. Give them the right support in the right places and they will go so far.

I have an abundance of people to thank in my journey with ADHD. My Mother who is my rock and still to this day puts me on the right path. My Father who taught me hard work and graft- and still does to this day; my brother who cultivated my very strange yet beautiful mind (sit still no, but boy, I am as sharp as a razor sometimes); my Grandparents and my Uncle Philip.

But last and not least my wonderful partner in crime, Becky- who I need to thank for being brash enough to say yes to me all that time ago. For being foolish enough to stay with me, and for loving me in a way I never thought I could be loved.

I hope you have enjoyed reading my story as much as I have writing it.

I have no doubt this publication will be a massive success. Dr Harpin is a lady I have no superlatives for. Her advice is impeccable. Her understanding immense and her dedication to the field of ADHD, long before I was born, amazing.

Remember, believe and have the faith that the light at the end of the tunnel is not just a silly phrase but an incredible possibility.

David Tompkinson

Chapter 1

ADHD: background and introduction

Val Harpin

ADHD can be defined simply as

'a developmentally inappropriate level of inattention and/or hyperactivity-impulsivity present before the age of 12 years that causes significant impairment'.

Diagnosing ADHD is, of course, much more complex than that sounds. Attention deficit hyperactivity disorder (ADHD) is a chronic, highly comorbid, neurodevelopmental disorder (Biederman et al. 1991; Kadesjo & Gillberg 2001; Yoshimasum et al. 2012) that typically presents with symptoms of inattention, impulsivity and hyperactivity and may have a profound impact on the individual and their family (Pliszka 1998; Harpin 2005; Biederman & Faraone 2005; Faraone et al. 2006; Loe & Feldman 2007).

This book will take a practical but evidence-based look at the diagnosis and management of ADHD in children and young people.

The evolution of the concept of ADHD

The use of the diagnosis of ADHD has been the subject of considerable controversy and debate. Even now, ADHD is seen, by some, as a new and invented disorder used by parents to explain the bad behaviour of their children. The National Institute for Health and Care Excellence (NICE) Guideline Development Group reviewed, in depth, the evidence that ADHD is a valid diagnostic construct, going back to the earliest literature and following the emergence of the concept and the supporting evidence. Their review and critique of the evidence is well worth reading (NICE 2008). The Group concluded that there was strong evidence for the clustering of inattentive and hyperactive-impulsive symptoms in both population and clinical samples and that ADHD should be viewed as one component of a group of neurodevelopmental problems that arises from shared aetiological influences. The data reviewed also evidenced that the cluster of symptoms consistent with ADHD persists over time and causes significant impairment.

There have, in fact, been descriptions of children with ADHD throughout history. The first example of a medical description of a disorder that appears to be similar to ADHD was given by Scottish physician Sir Alexander Crichton in 1798, when he described 'the incapacity of attending with a necessary degree of constancy to any one object'. Eminent British paediatrician Sir George Still published in the *Lancet* in 1902, describing children with a 'defect of moral control' (Still 1902). He stressed that inattention, impulsivity and hyperactivity played a major role and that the condition did not respond to punishment. Later, the idea of minimal brain damage was formed, although the symptoms were also seen in individuals with no apparent neurological damage. The evolution of the concept of ADHD is described in Box 1.1, and the diagnostic criteria from DSM-5 (American Psychiatric Association 2013) are discussed further in Chapter 3.

The International Classification of Diseases (ICD-10) (WHO) coding has been used in the UK and Europe. These criteria require symptoms to be present before the age of 7 years and to be of at least 6 months duration. The term 'hyperkinetic disorder' is used. The ICD criteria are currently under revision. Currently, the DSM criteria are most commonly used in research and in clinical practice and will be used here.

Box 1.1: Illustration of the evolution of the concept of ADHD from Still's description to the current American Psychiatric Association Diagnostic and Statistical Manual Version 5 (DSM-5)

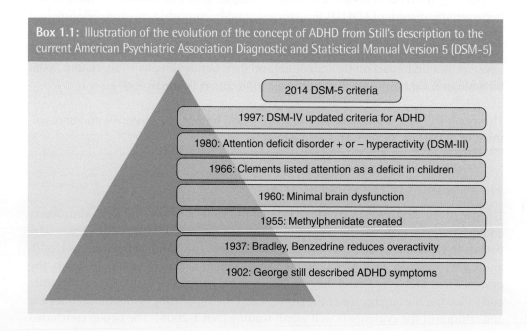

2014 DSM-5 criteria

1997: DSM-IV updated criteria for ADHD

1980: Attention deficit disorder + or – hyperactivity (DSM-III)

1966: Clements listed attention as a deficit in children

1960: Minimal brain dysfunction

1955: Methylphenidate created

1937: Bradley, Benzedrine reduces overactivity

1902: George still described ADHD symptoms

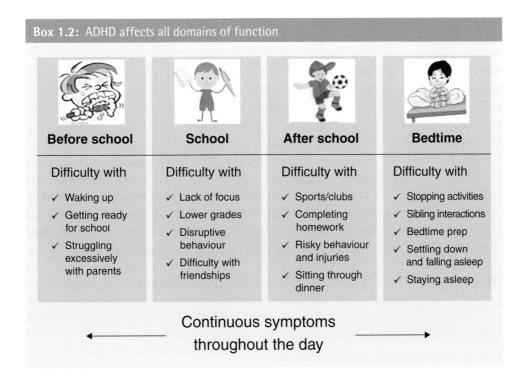

Box 1.2: ADHD affects all domains of function

Before school	School	After school	Bedtime
Difficulty with	Difficulty with	Difficulty with	Difficulty with
✓ Waking up ✓ Getting ready for school ✓ Struggling excessively with parents	✓ Lack of focus ✓ Lower grades ✓ Disruptive behaviour ✓ Difficulty with friendships	✓ Sports/clubs ✓ Completing homework ✓ Risky behaviour and injuries ✓ Sitting through dinner	✓ Stopping activities ✓ Sibling interactions ✓ Bedtime prep ✓ Settling down and falling asleep ✓ Staying asleep

Continuous symptoms
throughout the day

ADHD affects all aspects of an individual's life, as shown in Box 1.2.

Prevalence of ADHD

One of the major issues of controversy in the UK setting is the very high and variable prevalence rates for ADHD reported in the literature. ADHD is a common disorder. In the UK, The British Child and Adolescent Mental Health Survey (1999) carefully assessed 10 438 children between the ages of 5 and 15 years. The survey also included impairment in the diagnosis. This documented that 3.62% of boys and 0.85% of girls had ADHD (Ford et al. 2003).

A study in Newcastle in the UK that specifically addressed the role of impairment found that among 7- to 8-year-old children, 11.1% had the ADHD syndrome based on symptom count alone. When impairment was also taken into account, 6.7% had ADHD, with Children's Global Assessment Scale (C-GAS, measuring impairment) scores of less than 71, and only 4.2% had C-GAS scores of less than 61. When pervasiveness included both parent- and teacher-reported ADHD symptoms and the presence of psychosocial impairment, the prevalence fell further to 1.4%.

The more restricted ICD-10 diagnosis of 'hyperkinetic disorder' is naturally less common, with prevalence estimates of around 1.5% for boys of primary school age (McArdle et al. 2004).

In the international scientific literature, prevalence estimates for ADHD vary widely across studies. Polanczyk and colleagues (2007) undertook a systematic review of prevalence studies and concluded that the great majority of variability derived from the methods used, such as the way symptoms were measured and the exact definitions used. If this was taken into account there were relatively minor differences across the world, and the estimated ADHD worldwide, pooled prevalence was around 5.3%. The same authors published an update of this review in 2014 (Polanczyk et al. 2014). They concluded that the new meta-regression analyses confirmed that 'variability in ADHD prevalence estimates is mostly explained by methodological characteristics of the studies. In the past three decades, there has been no evidence to suggest an increase in the number of children in the community who meet criteria for ADHD when standardised diagnostic procedures are followed'.

Sometimes it is helpful to divide ADHD into three presentations:

- combined (50–75%)

- primarily inattentive (20–30%)

- primarily hyperactive-impulsive (<15%)

However, this division needs to be fluid, as one individual is likely to have difficulties within different symptom areas at different times in their development. Current presentation 'type' should therefore only be seen as descriptive at that point in time.

The male-to-female ratio is often quoted as 4:1 in children and adolescents, and this is probably true of those currently seen in clinics. However, more girls are now being referred as more is known about the different profile of the disorder in some girls (see Chapter 14). In adult life, the male-to-female ratio appears to be around 1:1.

Until relatively recently, ADHD was thought to be a childhood disorder that disappeared before adulthood, but what was actually occurring was a change in the symptom profile with development over time, in particular a decrease in the hyperactivity component (Box 1.3). Up to 85% of those diagnosed as children continue to be impaired by ADHD symptoms as adolescents (Gittelman et al. 1985; Weiss et al. 1985; Barkley et al. 1990; Biederman et al. 1996) and up to 60% in adulthood (Faraone et al. 2006).

Outcomes of ADHD

Children and adolescents with ADHD often have poor social skills, learning difficulties and disruptive behaviour, resulting in low self-esteem, difficult relationships and academic failure. Up to 30% of children with ADHD have an associated learning disorder of

---

Box 1.3: Symptom profile showing development over time

Preschool

Reduced play intensity
and duration
Motor restlessness
Hyperactive++
Impulsive

**Associated
problems
and implications**

✓ Developmental
  deficits

✓ Oppositional
  defiant behaviour

✓ Problems of social
  adaptation

Primary school age

Distractability

Motor restlessness

Impulsive and
disruptive behaviour

**Associated
problems and
implications**

✓ Specific learning
  disorders

✓ Aggressive behaviour

✓ Low self-esteem

✓ Repetition of classes/
  grades

✓ Rejection by peers

✓ Impaired family
  relationships

Adolescent

Persistent
inattention and
impulsivity

Reduction of motor
restlessness

Difficulty in planning
and organisation and
starting tasks and
sustaining effort

Associated problems

✓ Aggressive,
  antisocial and
  delinquent behaviour

✓ Alcohol and drug
  problems

✓ Emotional problems

✓ Accidents

---

reading, writing and/or mathematics (Biederman et al. 1991; Pliszka 1998), often requiring additional support in school and still resulting in poorer grades and a greater likelihood of repeating a school year when compared with controls (Loe & Feldman 2007).

Adolescents are at increased risk of suspension or expulsion (Frazier et al. 2007) and spend a shorter overall time in education (McGee et al. 1991). Young adults living with ADHD are more likely to have adverse psychiatric outcomes, including conduct disorder, antisocial, addictive and substance misuse disorders, mood and anxiety disorders (Biederman et al. 2006; Bussing et al. 2010). Indeed, those diagnosed in childhood have continued to show significantly worse educational, occupational, economic and social outcomes three decades after initial diagnosis compared with age-matched controls (Klein et al. 2012).

Barkley and colleagues followed a cohort of children diagnosed in Milwaukee, USA, from 1978 to 1980, and compared them with matched controls at an average age of 27 years. As found in other studies, over 60% of these individuals still had some symptoms of ADHD as adults. The ADHD cohort had significantly poorer educational outcomes, more learning disorders, and more psychiatric disorders, including oppositional defiant disorder, conduct disorder, depression, suicidal ideation and suicidal attempts, anxiety, eating disorders and substance misuse. These young adults also had more employment problems and workplace difficulties. In addition, the Milwaukee study showed an increase in motor vehicle accidents including fatalities, an increase in attendance at emergency departments, and a greater incidence of unplanned pregnancies.

A review using the Danish National register demonstrated that individuals with ADHD were more than twice as likely to die prematurely than those without ADHD (Dalsgaard et al. 2015).

There is therefore very clear evidence that ADHD merits diagnosis and treatment.

Proposed aetiologies

ADHD is a disorder with complex and multiple causes (Box 1.4).

Neurotransmitters and neuroanatomy

Within the brain, neurotransmitters transfer messages, and in individuals with ADHD this appears to be less effective in some regions of the brain, reducing the efficiency of some pathways in the brain. This is supported by the efficacy of medications that affect dopamine or noradrenaline transport. Systematic evidence also supports a role

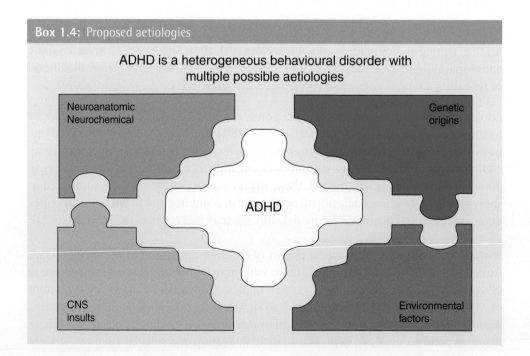

Box 1.4: Proposed aetiologies

ADHD is a heterogeneous behavioural disorder with multiple possible aetiologies

Neuroanatomic
Neurochemical

Genetic origins

ADHD

CNS insults

Environmental factors

Box 1.5: Functional circuits involved in the pathophysiology of ADHD

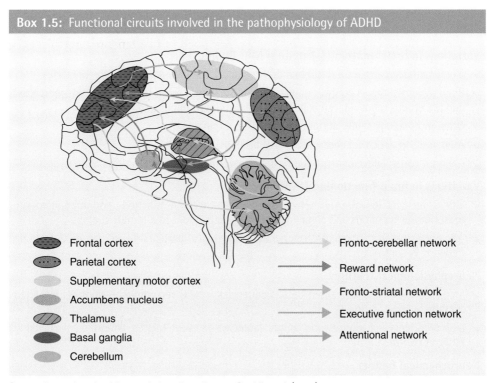

Frontal cortex	Fronto-cerebellar network
Parietal cortex	Reward network
Supplementary motor cortex	Fronto-striatal network
Accumbens nucleus	Executive function network
Thalamus	Attentional network
Basal ganglia	
Cerebellum	

Source: Reproduced, with permission, from Purper-Ouakil et al. (2011).

for other systems, including the serotonergic and cholinergic pathways. Purper-Ouakil has reviewed in detail the neurobiology of ADHD (Purper-Ouakil et al. 2011) and describes the circuits involved in the pathophysiology of ADHD (Box 1.5). Structural brain imaging studies have associated a number of structural abnormalities with ADHD in children and adolescents, including delayed cortical development, cortical thinning and reductions in the volume of grey and white matter, reduction in the volume of several regions of the brain, including the posterior inferior vermis, splenium of the corpus callosum, total and right cerebral volume, right caudate, right global pallidus, right anterior frontal region, cerebellum, temporal lobe and pulvinar (Nakao et al. 2011). Currently, none of these findings is helpful in diagnosis. Gogtay and colleagues (2004) elegantly describe the development of the brain from early childhood to young adult life. The areas related to ADHD, especially the frontal lobes, mature late in normal developmental patterns and it is estimated that this occurs even more slowly in young people with ADHD so that they are effectively functioning emotionally around 3 years behind their peers.

Cortese (2012) has provided an excellent review to outline 'What every clinician should know'. Table 1.1 summarises the main points he discusses.

Table 1.1   Anatomical, functional, neurophysiological, neurochemical and genetic correlates of ADHD

Variations in brain anatomy (structural MRI findings)

✓ Significant decrease in total cerebral and cerebellar volume compared with controls

✓ Brain abnormalities vs controls observed in frontostriatal areas, temporoparietal lobes, basal ganglia, corpus callosum, cerebellum, amygdala, hippocampus and thalamus

✓ Other morphological alterations, such as cortical thinning

✓ Alterations in structural connectivity (DTI findings)

✓ Aberrant cortical development and/or delayed normal cortical maturation

Variations in brain functioning (fMRI findings)

✓ Significant hypoactivation in networks related to executive functions, cognition, emotion, sensorimotor functions and compensatory hyperactivations in alternate regions

✓ Altered/perturbed pattern of functional connectivity, particularly in the default-mode network, vs controls

Neurophysiological features

✓ Increased theta, and decreased beta, frequencies in EEG recordings vs controls (elevated theta/beta power ratios)

✓ Less pronounced responses and longer latencies of event-related potentials, particularly P300, vs controls

Neurochemical factors

✓ Involvement of dopaminergic and adrenergic systems

  • Decreased availabilty of DA receptor isoforms and increased DAT binding vs controls

  • Current ADHD drug therapies block DA and NE reuptake and/or promote their release

✓ Serotonergic and cholinergic systems may also be involved

Genetic and environmental factors

✓ Heritability of ADHD: ~60–75%

✓ Involvement in ADHD of genes coding for bioforms of the DA raceptor, DA beta-hydroxylase, synaptosomal-associated protein 25, the serotonin transporter and the serotonin 1B receptor

✓ Pre-, peri- and post-natal environmental factors account for ~20–25% of the aetiology of ADHD

  • Most reliable associations with low birth weight/prematurity and exposure to maternal smoking in utero

✓ Likely contribution to ADHD aetiology of G x E interactions (epigenetic changes in gene expression caused by specific environmental factors)

Notes: ADHD, attention-deficit/hyperactivity disorder, DTI, diffusion tensor imaging EEG, electroencephalography; fMRI, functional MRI; G x E, gene–environment; MRI, magnetic resonance imaging.

Source: Reproduced, with permission, from Cortese (2012).

Genetics

ADHD runs in families. First-degree relatives of individuals with ADHD are two to eight times more likely to have ADHD than relatives of unaffected individuals (Faraone et al. 2005). There is at least a 50% chance that a child with ADHD will have at least one parent with ADHD and that a parent may have more than one child with ADHD. Exactly how and why ADHD is inherited has been the subject of much research, but is still unclear. Twin studies show high heritability rates of 71–90% for ADHD (Faraone et al. 2005). Heritability rates include genetic and gene–environment interplay, thus recognising the importance of environmental risks.

Importantly, adoption studies, where inherited and postnatal environmental effects are separated, also show a strong inherited contribution. Further studies are needed, however, looking particularly at those adopted at birth to remove any possible influence of early postnatal adversity.

Twin studies also demonstrate shared inherited factors with a wide range of neuro-developmental disorders, a strong argument for considering ADHD to be part of the group of neurodevelopmental disorders (as in DSM-5).

ADHD is also comorbid with several psychiatric and behavioural disorders, but there is a key difference in that some of these problems present later in development and could therefore be a consequence of having ADHD. Early onset conduct disorder is an exception to this (see Chapter 4, which describes coexisting conditions).

Early studies on the genetics of ADHD were candidate gene association studies. The most consistent candidate genes, after meta-analysis, were dopaminergic genes, serotonergic genes and the SNAP-25 gene, which is involved in neurotransmitter release, synaptic plasticity and axonal growth.

Later studies searched the genome for common DNA sequence variants, rare chromosomal structural variants, including copy number variants, which are subtle chromosomal deletions and duplications.

It is hoped, in the future, that genetic findings in ADHD might relate to the phenotype of ADHD and thereby help to tailor treatment more accurately to an individual. So far, there is insufficient replication of results, but there is a functional variant in the gene encoding the enzyme COMT (catechol-O-methyltransferase) with ADHD with conduct disorder. COMT is the primary mechanism for the breakdown of dopamine in the prefrontal cortex, and the gene variant increases the rate of dopamine breakdown.

More detail on genetic studies and the affect of environment are found in review articles by Thapar et al. (2013) and Gallo and Posner (2016).

Brain injury
Any injury to the brain predisposes an individual to ADHD. This may be due to accidental trauma, any cause of hypoxic brain injury (e.g. drowning or strangling), or infection (e.g. meningitis or encephalitis).

Preterm birth is known to increase the risk of all neurodevelopmental disorders, and rates of ADHD are significantly higher than in children born at term. In the Epicure study follow-up at the age of 11 years, ADHD inattentive type was found in 7.1% of those born preterm versus 0.7% in classmate controls. The incidence of ADHD combined type was also increased, at 4.4% versus 2.2% in controls (Kochar et al. 2009).

There is also an increased incidence of ADHD in individuals with epilepsy. These coexisting/comorbid conditions and how they affect management are considered further in Chapters 4 and 11.

Environmental factors
The environment in which an individual develops, particularly within the womb and in their early years, has a clear influence on the risk of having ADHD. The presence of social adversity also influences the course of the disorder and the response to treatment.

The interaction between the psychosocial environment and ADHD is complex, and the relationship between 'attachment disorder', emotional neglect and ADHD is difficult to unravel. The NICE Guideline Group was clear that the presence of attachment disorder should not preclude treatment for ADHD if diagnostic criteria are met (NICE 2008). Parenting style can clearly influence the degree of impairment, and the presence of maternal mental health problems such as depression and anxiety may also have some effect on vulnerable children. The interaction between genetic and environmental factors may be key. There is strong evidence of interaction between genetic and some environmental factors; for example, Kahn and colleagues (2003) demonstrated that being homozygous for the DAT 1 gene alone appears to have a minimal affect on the risk of ADHD, but the addition of prenatal exposure to maternal smoking significantly increases the risk (Box 1.6).

There appears to be a similar relationship with exposure to maternal alcohol and drugs in pregnancy.

For a systematic review of environmental, antenatal and early years risk factors see Latimer et al. (2012).

Relationship with other conditions
There is an increased risk of ADHD in several inherited disorders, such as neurofibromatosis and fragile X. ADHD is also more common in individuals with chronic neurological

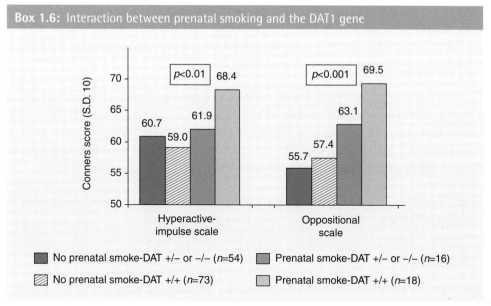

Box 1.6: Interaction between prenatal smoking and the DAT1 gene

Source: Adapted, with permission, from Kahn et al. (2003).

illness such as epilepsy or metabolic problems (e.g. phenylketonuria [PKU]), with Williams syndrome, hyperthyroidism, tuberous sclerosis, XYY, XXY, fragile X, 22q11 microdeletion syndrome, cyanotic congenital heart disease and following some medical treatments such as cerebral irradiation or anticonvulsants.

All of these factors need to be considered carefully during diagnostic assessment and ongoing management.

The cost of ADHD

We have considered some of the emotional and financial costs to those with ADHD and their families.

The costs to society of managing ADHD are also high, in part as a result of the associated problems, including self-harm, increased road traffic (and other) accidents, substance misuse, delinquency, anxiety states and academic underachievement. Those with other chronic conditions alongside ADHD, such as asthma, often have difficulty following regular treatment regimes, and the outcome is an increased need for services. There is also a cost from the necessary absence from employment of carers of children with ADHD. Although exact healthcare costs for individuals with ADHD are difficult to quantify, evidence from the UK and the USA shows the annual medical costs for someone with ADHD to be more than twice those of someone without ADHD. There are also cost implications for education services, social care and the justice system. For further information see a useful review by Beecham (2014).

Currently in the UK, ADHD is most commonly diagnosed between the ages of 6 and 12 years (McCarthy et al. 2012). This is likely to be similar across Europe. The long-term impact that untreated or poorly treated ADHD can have on the individual with ADHD, their family and, importantly, their life chances, is profound. Thus, optimising the support these children, young people and adults and their families receive is paramount.

In the following chapters, current best practice in diagnosis and management will be considered further.

References

American Psychiatric Association (2013) *Diagnostic and statistical manual of mental disorders,* 5th edn. Arlington, VA: American Psychiatric Association.

Barkley RA, Fischer M, Edelbrock CS, Smallish L (1990) The adolescent outcome of hyperactive children diagnosed by research criteria: I. An 8-year prospective follow-up study. *J Am Acad Child Adolesc Psychiatry* 29(4): 546–557.

Beecham J (2014) Annual Research Review. Child and adolescent mental health interventions: A review of progress in economic studies across different disorders. *J Child Psychol Psychiatry* 55(6): 714–732, doi:10.1111/jcpp.12216.

Biederman J, Newcorn J, Sprich S. (1991) Comorbidity of attention deficit hyperactivity disorder with conduct, depressive, anxiety and other disorders. *Am J Psychiatry* 148(5): 564–577.

Biederman J, Faraone S, Milberger S et al. (1996) Predictors of persistence and remission of ADHD into adolescence: Results from a four-year prospective follow-up study. *J Am Acad Child Adolesc Psychiatry* 35(3): 343–351.

Biederman J, Faraone SV (2005) Attention-deficit hyperactivity disorder. *Lancet* 366(9481): 237–248.

Biederman J, Monuteaux MC, Mick E et al. (2006) Young adult outcome of attention deficit hyperactivity disorder: A controlled 10-year follow-up study. *Psychol Med* 36(2): 167–179.

Bussing R, Mason DM, Bell L, Porter P, Garvan C (2010) Adolescent outcomes of childhood attention-deficit/hyperactivity disorder in diverse community sample. *J Am Acad Child Adolesc Psychiatry* 49(6): 595–605.

Cortese S (2012) The neurobiology and genetics of attention- deficit/hyperactivity disorder (ADHD): What every clinician should know. *J Eur Paediatr Neurol Soc* 16: 422–433, doi:10.1016/j.ejpn.2012.01.09.

Dalsgaard S, Østergaard S, Leckman J, Mortensen P, Pedersen M (2015) Mortality in children, adolescents, and adults with attention deficit hyperactivity disorder: A nationwide cohort study. *Lancet* 385(9983): 2190–2196, doi:10.1016/S0140-6736(14)61684-6.

Faraone SV, Perlis RH, Doyle AE et al. (2005) Molecular genetics of attention-deficit/hyperactivity disorder. *Biol Psychiatry* 57(11): 1313–1323, doi:10.1016/j.biopsych.2004.11.024.

Faraone SV, Biederman J, Mick E (2006) The age-dependent decline of attention deficit hyperactivity disorder: a meta-analysis of follow-up studies. *Psychol Med* 36(2): 159–165.

Ford T, Goodman R, Meltzer H (2003) The British Child and Adolescent Mental Health Survey 1999: The prevalence of DSM-IV disorders. *J Am Acad Child Adolesc. Psychiatry* 42: 1203–1211.

Frazier TW, Youngstrom EA, Glutting JJ, Watkins MW (2007) ADHD and achievement: meta-analysis of the child, adolescent, and adult literatures and a concomitant study with college students. *J Learn Disabil* 40(1): 465.

Gallo E, Posner J (2016) Attention-deficit hyperactivity disorder 1. Moving towards causality in attention-deficit hyperactivity disorder: Overview of neural and genetic mechanisms. *Lancet Psychiatry* 3(6), 555–567, doi:10.1016/S2215-0366(16)00096-1.

Gittelman R, Mannuzza S, Shenker R, Bonagura N (1985) Hyperactive boys almost grown up. I. Psychiatric status. *Arch Gen Psychiatry* 42(10): 937–947.

Gogtay N, Giedd JN, Lusk L et al. (2004) Dynamic mapping of human cortical development during childhood through early adulthood. *Proc Natl Acad Sci USA* 101(21): 8174–8179, doi:10.1073/pnas.0402680101.

Harpin VA (2005) The effect of ADHD on the life of an individual, their family, and community from preschool to adult life. *Arch Dis Child* 90(Suppl. 1): i2–i7.

Kadesjo B, Gillberg C (2001) The comorbidity of ADHD in the general population of Swedish school-age children. *J Child Psychol Psychiatry* 42(4): 487–492.

Kahn J, Khoury J, Nichols WC, Lanphear BP (2003) Role of dopamine transporter genotype and maternal prenatal smoking in childhood hyperactive-impulsive, inattentive and oppositional behaviors. *J Pediatr* 143(1): 104–110.

Klein RG, Mannuzza S, Olazagasti MA et al. (2012) Clinical and functional outcome of childhood attention-deficit/hyperactivity disorder 33 years later. *Arch Gen Psychiatry* 69(12): 1295–1303.

Kochhar P, Johnson S, Hollis C, Marlow N (2009) Psychiatric and behavioural disorders at 11 years of age in children born extremely preterm (the Epicure Study). *Arch Dis Child* 94: A1–A8.

Latimer K, Wilson P, Kemp J et al. (2012) Disruptive behaviour disorders: A systematic review of environmental, antenatal and early years risk factors. *Child Care Health Dev* 38(5): 611–628, doi:10.1111/j.1365-2214.2012.01366.x.

Loe IM, Feldman HM (2007) Academic and educational outcome of children with ADHD. *J Pediatr Psychol.* 32(6): 643–654.

McCarthy S, Wilton L, Murray ML, Hodgkins P, Asherson P, Wong IC (2012) The epidemiology of pharmacologically treated attention deficit hyperactivity disorder (ADHD) in children, adolescents and adults in UK primary care. *BMC Pediatr* 12: 78.

McArdle P, Prosser J, Kolvin I (2004) Prevalence of psychiatric disorder: With and without psychosocial impairment. *Eur Child Adolesc Psychiatry* 13(6): 347–353.

McGee R, Partridge F, Williams S, Silva PA (1991) A twelve-year follow-up of preschool hyperactive children. *J Am Acad Child Adolesc Psychiatry* 30(2): 224–232.

Nakao T, Radua J, Rubia K et al. (2011) Gray matter volume abnormalities in ADHD: Voxel-based meta-analysis exploring the effects of age and stimulant medication. *Am J Psychiatry* 168: 1154–1163.

NICE (2008) *Attention deficit hyperactivity disorder: Diagnosis and management. NICE Clinical Guidelines* [CG72], https://www.nice.org.uk/guidance/cg72.

Pliszka SR (1998) Comorbidity of attention-deficit/hyperactivity disorder with psychiatry disorder: An overview. *J Clin Psychiatry* 59(Suppl. 7): 50–58.

Polanczyk G, de Lima MS, Horta BL, Biederman J, Rohde LA (2007) The worldwide prevalence of ADHD: A systematic review and metaregression analysis. *Am J Psychiatry* 164(6): 942–948.

Polanczyk GV, Willcutt EG, Salum GA, Kieling C, Rohde LA (2014) ADHD prevalence estimates across three decades: an updated systematic review and meta-regression analysis. *Int J Epidemiol* 43(2): 434–442, doi:10.1093/ije/dyt261.

Purper-Ouakil D, Ramoz N, Lepagnol-Bestel AM, Gorwood P, Simonneau M (2011) Neurobiology of attention deficit/hyperactivity disorder. *Pediatr Res* 69(5): 69Re76R.

Still G (1902) Some abnormal psychical conditions in children: The Goulstonian lectures. *Lancet* 1: 1008–1012.

Thapar A, Cooper M, Eyre O, Langley K (2013) Practitioner Review: What have we learnt about the causes of ADHD? *J Child Psychol Psychiatry* 54(1): 3–16, doi:10.1111/j.1469-7610.2012.02611.x.

Weiss G, Hechtman L, Milroy T, Perlman T (1985) Psychiatric status of hyperactives as adults: A controlled prospective 15-year follow-up of 63 hyperactive children. *J Am Acad Child Psychiatry* 24(2): 211–220.

WHO www.who.int/classifications/icd/icdonlineversions/en/.

Yoshimasum K, Barbaresi WJ, Colligan RC et al. (2012) Childhood ADHD is strongly associated with a broad range of psychiatric disorders during adolescence: A population-based birth cohort study. *J Child Psychol Psychiatry* 53(10): 1036–1043.

Chapter 2

Referral: how to inform, educate and support referrers

Val Harpin

Despite the fact that rates of diagnosis of ADHD have risen significantly in recent years, current UK prevalence figures still suggest that ADHD is under recognised (NICE 2008). The numbers have risen from an estimate of 0.5 per 1000 children diagnosed in the UK 30 years ago (Taylor 1986), to more than 3 per 1000 receiving medication for ADHD in the late 1990s (NICE 2006). The prevalence of pharmaco-logical treatment of ADHD increased further until 2008 (McCarthy et al. 2012). The increase included more adults and more girls with ADHD. Healthcare Improvement Scotland published their report of ADHD in Scotland in 2012 and concluded that 'the diagnostic rate for ADHD in school-aged children in Scotland falls far short of what we would expect'.

In 2013, The Care Quality Commission raised concerns that prescriptions for ADHD medications had risen by 50% in the previous 6 years. However, the evidence is that in the UK the incidence of ADHD diagnosis still remains lower than the expected incidence of the diagnosis of even severe ADHD.

It is also clear that there is often a long delay before referral and finally diagnosis take place. A naturalistic study (a study in which the researcher observes and records what is actually happening, in this case in clinical services, without influencing it) in Europe (ADORE) found that diagnosis of ADHD was confirmed on average around 4 years after symptoms were first recognised (Preuss et al. 2006).

How do we try to ensure that the children who need ADHD services are referred in a timely fashion? And that referral of large numbers of children who do not have ADHD is avoided?

Services are already stretched by the rising level of referrals, so, ideally, referral for assessment should target those most in need and not include large numbers of children and young people who on assessment do not have ADHD. Sensitive and yet specific referral criteria for ADHD are, however, not easy to find.

Who makes referrals?

Most referrals are from general practitioners (GPs) at the instigation of parents or education-based professionals. Some assessment services also accept referrals directly from educational psychologists and special educational needs coordinators.

These professionals need a basic understanding of ADHD and what symptoms they should be looking for. The training of GPs and indeed most other doctors includes only a little on ADHD, and education professionals often have very little training on special educational needs overall. Increasingly they will have learnt by teaching children with the diagnosis. It is vital for optimal support for children and young people with ADHD and their families that health and education teams work together and take every opportunity to meet and discuss individual children and ADHD and comorbid difficulties as a whole.

Which children should be referred?

Think about each child or young person described below.

Think also about any other information you might like before referral and whether the ADHD Assessment Team should see them.

Connor, aged 8 years

- His school and mother are very concerned.

- Connor has a long history of active 'silly' behaviour.

- There is a complex family history. Connor's father has had problems with the police. He no longer lives in the family, but Connor stays with his paternal grandmother alternate weekends and sees his father then. Connor has an older sister, aged 17 years, who has a new baby and lives with her partner in the house.

- Connor struggles academically. His teacher thinks he has specific learning difficulties but that he is significantly under-achieving for his potential.

- He has few friends and spends time with older boys.

- He often plays on his X box until after midnight.

- Connor already misses school frequently.

- His language development appears good, but he swears incessantly.

Alex, aged 5 years

- Alex's parents and school are very concerned.

- He is the only child of two university lecturers.

- He has always been active and a 'real boy'.

- Alex seems very bright but will not engage with teachers.

- He seems angry all the time.

- Alex never stops day or night, and he and his parents are getting little sleep.

- He struggles to make friends. He has never been invited to a classmate's birthday party, and his grandparents will not have him to stay.

Sophie, aged 14 years

- Sophie lives with her parents and younger sister.

- She managed well in her small local primary school and left with average results.

- Since moving to secondary school, aged 11 years, things have been going downhill, academically and socially.

- Recently, her parents found out that Sophie was drinking regularly, sometimes before school.

- Her mother was devastated to discover fresh scarring on Sophie's left forearm.

- Sophie's parents are confused and angry.

- Now Sophie is tearful and desperate because a pregnancy test is positive.

Arron, aged 16 years

- Arron was referred by a youth worker and arrives in your clinic in handcuffs accompanied by the police.

- There is a long history of minor theft and disturbance.

- The current arrest is for carrying a knife and stealing a car.

- Arron has been in and out of care. His mother is a long-term drug user. He is currently living with his caring but elderly grandmother.

- Arron uses cannabis daily, sometimes with friends and sometimes alone.

- Arron seems 'bright' but he is out of school and has no hope of a job.

Ethan, aged 3 years

- Ethan never stops, day or night.

- His mother is a single parent with little support.

- He has two half siblings aged 18 months and 5 years.

- He was born preterm at 28 weeks gestation.

- Generally, his development has been within average, but he has delayed language and poor play skills.

- The nursery he attends is very committed to Ethan, but they struggle with his high activity levels and impulsive behaviour and are very concerned.

- Ethan recently bit and hit a girl in nursery and this prompted the referral.

Aidan, aged 8 years

- Aidan was adopted at the age of 3 years.

- His adoptive parents are both lawyers aged 40 years.

- There was a history of heavy maternal alcohol consumption in pregnancy, and also drug use.

- Aidan has problems with language development and was slow to develop toileting skills. He still wets the bed.

- He 'seems bright' but struggles academically.

- At school, friendships are not sustained, but he does enjoy meeting his new cousins.

- School suggest to his parents that they should request assessment of possible ADHD.

Max, aged 10 years

- Max has moderate learning disability secondary to a chromosomal anomaly.

- He attends a special resource in a primary school. His father feels he is not making the progress he should and has been to see his teacher.

• The teacher expresses concerns about poor concentration, but does not know if this is solely due to his learning disability.

All of those descriptions, and indeed many more, could indicate ADHD. None, however, is enough to make a diagnosis alone.

What can be done before specialist assessment? (Box 2.1)

A great deal more information is required as part of the diagnostic assessment process (see Chapter 3). However, before referral, if possible, there should always be discussion between the family and the school or nursery. Information from a teacher to support referral is helpful to try to direct families to the most appropriate support.

Remember, also, that it is very common for the core problems of ADHD in children to present together with other developmental impairments and/or mental health problems. There are many non-specific problems that are very common in children with ADHD, but may also masquerade as ADHD. Information about noncompliant behaviour, motor tics, aggression, unpopularity with peers, temper tantrums, clumsiness, literacy and other learning problems and immature or disordered language and social skills is

---

Box 2.1: Information to include when making a referral

Any referral should be accompanied by as much information as possible on the following:

✓ A brief description of the family's concerns, with particular reference to examples of poor concentration and hyperactive/impulsive behaviours
✓ Details of the family composition and any history of family mental health problems
✓ Information from school about academic performance, behaviour and peer relationships
✓ Past medical history
✓ Developmental history:
  • Delay in any areas
  • Motor coordination difficulties
  • Social skills difficulties
  • Specific learning difficulties
✓ History of mental health difficulties:
  • Anxiety
  • Low self-esteem/depression
  • Self harm
  • Substance misuse
✓ Any concerns about hearing or vision
✓ Details of any other involved professionals

helpful. Some teams use a structured pre-assessment proforma to gather information like this to inform and direct referrals.

Some assessment teams send out ADHD-specific or broadband questionnaires (e.g. Conners or Strengths and difficulties questionnaires) before children are seen. This may be useful as part of the assessment process, but may also be used to redirect referrals if not supportive of ADHD as the primary diagnosis.

Education professionals and primary-care health professionals (e.g. GPs or school nurses) should consider offering families written information about ADHD or website addresses if they are confident in the information source (see Appendix 1 for suggestions).

There is often a significant wait before children and young people can be seen by specialist child and adolescent psychiatry or psychology teams (CAMHS in the UK) or paediatric/child development teams. Ideally, support should be offered to families during that time. First, consideration should be given to referral for behaviour management advice if the family have not yet tried this. At this point this will most probably be a non-specific programme such as Webster Stratton (incredibleyears.com) or Triple P (triplep.net). There is some evidence that such programmes can be helpful (NICE 2008) although this is not always the case. Current NICE Guidelines recommend behavioural management as the first-line treatment for mild and moderate ADHD, but a meta-analysis of their efficacy may cause review of this recommendation in the future in some cases (Sonuga-Barke et al. 2013). Ideally, behavioural management programmes should be eight to ten sessions long, run by trained facilitators and ADHD specific, but many areas cannot currently offer this, especially prior to full assessment.

If ADHD is strongly suspected, it is vital to inform facilitators of any general parent management programme of this and to reassure the family that developing clear behaviour management techniques, while sometimes difficult and even apparently unsuccessful for such children and families, is a vital part of helping their child. Again, if ADHD is strongly suspected, it may be helpful, while being clear that the diagnosis has not been confirmed, to refer families to local or national support groups (see Appendix 1).

Summary

- Raising awareness of ADHD among health, education and social care professionals and with families will facilitate appropriate, timely referral.

- Prior to formal assessment, the collection of relevant information from home and school can be used to direct referrals correctly.

> • Before a diagnosis is confirmed, families may be helped by access to general behaviour management advice, information about ADHD and how it can affect children and young people, and contact with parent support groups.

References

Healthcare Improvement Scotland (2012) *Attention deficit and hyperkinetic disorders services over Scotland. Final Report November 2012.* Healthcare Improvement Scotland; available at http://www.healthcareimprovementscotland.org/our_work/mental_health/adhd_service_improvement/stage_3_adhd_final_report.aspx.

McCarthy S, Asherson P, Coghill D (2009) Attention-deficit hyperactivity disorder: Treatment discontinuation in adolescents and young adults. *Br J Psychiatry* 194(3): 273–277.

McCarthy S, Wilton L, Murray ML, Hodgkins P, Asherson P, Wong ICK (2012) The epidemiology of pharmacologically treated attention deficit hyperactivity disorder (ADHD) in children, adolescents and adults in UK primary care. *BMC Pediatr* 12: 78.

NICE (2006) *Methylphenidate, atomoxetine and dexamfetamine for attention deficit hyperactivity disorder (ADHD) in children and adolescents,* Technology appraisal guidance TA98.

NICE (2008) *Attention deficit hyperactivity disorder: Diagnosis and management.*

NICE Clinical Guidelines [CG72], https://www.nice.org.uk/guidance/cg72.

Preuss U, Ralston SJ, Baldursson G et al.; ADORE Study Group (2006) Study design, baseline patient characteristics and intervention in a cross-cultural framework: Results from the ADORE study. *Eur Child Adolesc Psychiatry* 15(Suppl. 1): I4–14, doi:10.1007/s00787-006-1002-0.

Sonuga-Barke EJS, Brandeis D, Cortese S et al. and the European ADHD Guidelines Group (2013) Nonpharmacological interventions for ADHD: Systematic review and meta-analyses of randomized controlled trials of dietary and psychological treatments. *Am J Psychiatry* 170(3): 275–289, doi:10.1176/appi.ajp.2012.12070991.

Taylor E (1986) Overactivity, hyperactivity and hyperkinesis: Problems and prevalence. In: Taylor E, editor. *The overactive child: Clinics in developmental medicine,* no. 97. London, Oxford: Mac Keith Press & Blackwell.

Chapter 3

Diagnostic assessment: a step-by-step approach

Val Harpin

We continue to have concerns regarding schooling. He is a lucky boy, taught in a class of 11, with extra support for English and maths. School are fabulously supportive and in the main receptive to anything that may assist Jamie.

Jamie is in Y4 probably working at Y1 level, he continues to struggle with writing, spelling and very much with maths, underpinning all of this is his lack of ability to concentrate, his butterfly mind means very little is retained or understood.

Jamie manages to remain seated in the classroom on the whole, tries not to shout out and interrupt, but it seems much of his energy is spent doing the right thing, not learning.

Friendships continue to be difficult for Jamie because of impulsive behaviours, too much physical contact – being too much in other childrens' faces, intolerance and, occasionally at school, hitting and kicking, despite him realising this is unacceptable behaviour.

(Exert from an email written by Jamie's mother to inform
his ADHD assessment)

The timely and accurate diagnosis of ADHD is essential to providing much needed support to children and families. Evidence of the benefits of long-term treatment has not always seemed robust, but the implications for individual children, young people and their families is clear to clinicians in the field. A thorough systematic review of the outcomes of ADHD published in 2012 by Shaw et al. is useful reading. They reviewed outcome data from 351 studies in nine major areas: academic achievement, antisocial behaviour, driving, non-medicinal drug use/addictive behaviour, obesity, occupation, service use, self-esteem and social function outcomes. The review concluded that without treatment, people with ADHD had poorer long-term outcomes in all categories compared with people without ADHD, and that treatment for ADHD improved long-term outcomes compared with untreated ADHD, although not usually to outcome levels of those without ADHD.

There are also, however, implications of mis- or over-diagnosis, including labelling, stigma and potentially inappropriate long-term treatment with medications that may carry significant side effects.

Services that provide assessment for possible ADHD vary widely. Most involve either a child and adolescent psychiatrist or a specialist paediatrician, and multidisciplinary teams will involve a range of clinicians including psychologists, specialist nurses and other therapists. Optimal diagnosis and support will also involve close working with education and social care professionals and the use of voluntary agency input.

This chapter describes, step by step, the likely components of an assessment process. Which professional undertakes which part of an assessment process will vary from team to team. An effective team will contain or have easy access to all the relevant competencies.

There is no simple 'test' for ADHD. The diagnostic assessment of a child or young person who may have ADHD involves the careful collection and collation of information from home, from school, possibly from other carers (e.g. from afterschool clubs or leisure activities) and ideally a structured observation. This information is then interpreted using standard criteria, usually those from DSM-5 (Boxes 3.1 and 3.2) (American Psychiatric Association 2013).

At least six of the nine inattention symptoms and six of the nine hyperactive-impulsive symptoms must be present. The clinician must interpret what constitutes 'often'. This interpretation requires knowledge of the range of normal childhood behaviour and information about this child/young person from as many sources as possible.

To make a diagnosis of ADHD the following criteria must also be met:

- Some hyperactive-impulsive or inattentive symptoms that caused impairment were present before the age of 12 years (previously 7 years in DSM-IV but increased to 12 in DSM-5).

- Some impairment from symptoms is present in two or more settings, e.g. at school and at home.

- There is clear evidence of significant impairment in social and/or school functioning.

- Symptoms must not be solely attributable to other mental disorders, illnesses or environmental factors.

Box 3.1: DSM-5 Criteria for ADHD

Attention–Deficit/Hyperactivity Disorder

Diagnostic Criteria

A. A persistent pattern of inattention and/or hyperactivity-impulsivity that interferes with functioning or development, as characterized by (1) and/or (2):

✓ **Inattention:** Six (or more) of the following symptoms have persisted for at least 6 months to a degree that is inconsistent with developmental level and that negatively impacts directly on social and academic/occupational activities:

Note: The symptoms are not solely a manifestation of oppositional behavior, defiance, hostility, or failure to understand tasks or instructions. For older adolescents and adults (age 17 and older), at least five symptoms are required.

- Often fails to give close attention to details or makes careless mistakes in schoolwork, at work, or during other activities (e.g., overlooks or misses details, work is inaccurate).
- Often has difficulty sustaining attention in tasks or play activities (e.g., has difficulty remaining focused during lectures, conversations, or lengthy reading).
- Often does not seem to listen when spoken to directly (e.g., mind seems elsewhere, even in the absence of any obvious distraction).
- Often does not follow through on instructions and fails to finish schoolwork, chores, or duties in the workplace (e.g., starts tasks but quickly loses focus and is easily sidetracked).
- Often has difficulty organizing tasks and activities (e.g., difficulty managing sequential tasks; difficulty keeping materials and belongings in order; messy, disorganized work; has poor time management; fails to meet deadlines).
- Often avoids, dislikes, or is reluctant to engage in tasks that require sustained mental effort (e.g., schoolwork or homework; for older adolescents and adults, preparing reports, completing forms, reviewing lengthy papers).
- Often loses things necessary for tasks or activities (e.g., school materials, pencils, books, tools, wallets, keys, paperwork, eyeglasses, mobile telephones).
- Is often easily distracted by extraneous stimuli (for older adolescents and adults, may include unrelated thoughts).
- Is often forgetful in daily activities (e.g., doing chores, running errands; for older adolescents and adults, returning calls, paying bills, keeping appointments).

✓ **Hyperactivity and impulsivity:** Six (or more) of the following symptoms have persisted for at least 6 months to a degree that is inconsistent with developmental level and that negatively impacts directly on social and academic/occupational activities.

Note: The symptoms are not solely a manifestation of oppositional behavior, defiance, hostility, or a failure to understand tasks or instructions. For older adolescents and adults (age 17 and older), at least five symptoms are required.

- Often fidgets with or taps hands or feet or squirms in seat.
- Often leaves seat in situations when remaining seated is expected (e.g., leaves his or her place in the classroom, in the office or other workplace, or in other situations that require remaining in place).

> **Box 3.1:** Continued
>
> - Often runs about or climbs in situations where it is inappropriate. (**Note**: In adolescents or adults, may be limited to feeling restless.)
> - Often unable to play or engage in leisure activities quietly.
> - Is often 'on the go', acting as if 'driven by a motor' (e.g., is unable to be or uncomfortable being still for extended time, as in restaurants, meetings; may be experienced by others as being restless or difficult to keep up with).
> - Often talks excessively.
> - Often blurts out an answer before a questions has been completed (e.g., completes people's sentences; cannot wait for turn in conversation).
> - Often has difficulty waiting his or her turn (e.g., while waiting in line).
> - Often interrupts or intrudes on others (e.g., butts into conversations, games, or activities; may start using other people's things without asking or receiving permission; for adolescents and adults, may intrude into or take over what others are doing).

Source: Adapted from DSM-5 (2013).
Reprinted with permission from the Diagnostic and Statistical Manual of Mental Disorders, Fifth Edition, (Copyright © 2013). American Psychiatric Association. All Rights Reserved.

> **Box 3.2:** Additional information to assess the DSM-5 Criteria
>
> B. Several inattentive or hyperactive-impulsive symptoms were present prior to age 12 years.
>
> C. Several inattentive or hyperactive-impulsive symptoms are present in two or more settings (e.g., at home, school, or work; with friends or relatives; in other activities).
>
> D. There is clear evidence that the symptoms interfere with, or reduce the quality of, social, academic, or occupational functioning.
>
> E. The symptoms do not occur exclusively during the course of schizophrenia or another psychotic disorder and are not better explained by another mental disorder (e.g., mood disorder, anxiety disorder, dissociative disorder, personality disorder, substance intoxication or withdrawal).
>
> *Specify* whether:
>
> **314.01 (F90.2) Combined presentation:** If both Criterion A1 (inattention) and Criterion A2 (hyperactivity-impulsivity) are met for the past 6 months.
>
> **314.00 (F90.0) Predominantly inattentive presentation:** If Criterion A1 (inattention) is met but Criterion A2 (hyperactivity-impulsivity) is not met for the past 6 months.
>
> **314.01 (F90.1) Predominantly hyperactive/impulsive presentation:** If Criterion A2 (hyperactivity-impulsivity) is met and Criterion A1 (inattention) is not met for the past 6 months.
>
> *Specify* if:
>
> **In partial remission:** When full criteria were previously met, fewer than the full criteria have been met for the past 6 months, and the symptoms still result in impairment in social, academic, or occupational functioning.

> **Box 3.2:** Continued
>
> *Specify* current severity:
>
> **Mild:** Few, if any, symptoms in excess of those required to make the diagnosis are present, and symptoms result in no more than minor impairments in social or occupational functioning.
>
> **Moderate:** Symptoms or functional impairment between 'mild' and 'severe" are present.
>
> **Severe:** Many symptoms in excess of those required to make the diagnosis, or several symptoms that are particularly severe, are present, or the symptoms result in marked impairment in social or occupational functioning.

Source: Adapted from DSM-5 (2013).
Reprinted with permission from the Diagnostic and Statistical Manual of Mental Disorders, Fifth Edition, (Copyright © 2013). American Psychiatric Association. All Rights Reserved.

ICD-10 hyperkinetic disorder

The International Classification of Mental and Behavioural Disorders, 10th revision (ICD-10) medical classification system was developed by the World Health Organisation (www.who.int/classifications/icd/icdonlineversions/en/). ICD-10 uses the term hyperkinetic disorder (HKD), which is defined as a persistent and severe impairment of psychological development characterised by

- early onset (<6 years)

- overactive, poorly modulated behaviour

- marked inattention

- lack of persistent task involvement

- pervasiveness over situations (e.g. home and school) and persistence over time of these behavioural characteristics

- exclusion of a diagnosis of anxiety disorders, mood affective disorders, pervasive developmental disorders and schizophrenia.

HKD should only be diagnosed if these symptoms are excessive for the child's age, cognitive ability and situation.

Impairment

Impairment is a continuum and therefore not always easy to quantify. Box 3.3 shows the NICE Guideline Group's (2008) suggestions of areas where relevant impairment may be present.

Box 3.3: Assessing areas of impairment

In children and young people

Impairment in multiple domains including home and school where the level appropriate to the child's chronological and mental age has not been reached:

✓ Self-care (in eating, hygiene and so on); travelling independently

✓ Making and keeping friends

✓ Achieving in school

✓ Forming positive relationships with other family members

✓ Developing a positive self-image

✓ Avoiding criminal activity

✓ Avoiding substance misuse

✓ Maintaining emotional states free of excessive anxiety and unhappiness understanding and avoiding common hazards

In later adolescence and adult life

The range of possible impairments:

✓ Occupational underachievement

✓ Disputes in the workplace

✓ Dangerous driving

✓ Difficulties in carrying out daily activities such as shopping

✓ Organising household tasks

✓ Making and keeping friends

✓ In intimate relationships (e.g. excessive disagreement and frequent break-ups)

✓ With child care

Source: Adapted from NICE (2008).

In clinical practice, impairment can only be assessed by taking all the available evidence into account and referencing this with the clinician's knowledge of the range of average in the population.

The assessment process (Box 3.4) is designed to elicit and assess core symptoms, coexisting difficulties and resulting impairment.

History

Obtaining and recording a clear history is key to the accurate assessment of ADHD. Every clinician should develop a format for gathering the initial history to ensure that all relevant areas are covered. Some teams use a proforma to ensure that nothing is missed out and so that information is recorded in a format that can easily be referred to at a later date by the original and other clinicians. There are structured interviews

---

Box 3.4: The assessment process

The clinical interview

✓ Current concerns

✓ Past difficulties

✓ Developmental history

✓ Medical history including birth history

✓ Medication history

✓ Home environment

✓ Family history including parental/carer physical and mental health

✓ School life

✓ Sleep

✓ Coexisting neurodevelopmental/mental health difficulties

Other information

✓ Physical examination

✓ Possible investigation

✓ Observation: clinic/home/school

✓ Additional school information

✓ Questionnaires

✓ Computerised tests

✓ Bringing it all together

✓ Agreeing a diagnosis

---

available, but these are very lengthy and, although they are essential in research, they are seldom used in clinical practice.

The interview should include the main carer and, if the child/young person has two carers both carers' views need to be sought if at all possible. This may be two parents living with the child, a parent and step parent, two parents who live apart but both have access, adoptive parents, other family members or a long-term foster carer. Involving all relevant carers is helpful not only to gather accurate information to aid diagnosis but also, if ADHD is found to be present, it helps to have all parents/carers on board and involved in management decisions, particularly when discussing the need or otherwise for medication.

Current concerns

Always start by listening to the family's current concerns. This gives them a chance to explain why they and/or the school feel their son or daughter needs to be assessed and to explain what they hope to achieve by coming to the service. Use this opportunity to ask follow-up questions to cover the overall picture but ensure you have listened first.

Always try to elicit positives about the child or young person and things that go well for the family, as well as hearing about the negatives. Often, families have waited a long time to have the opportunity to talk to someone about their worries and they may focus totally on their negative experiences if you do not ask.

The concerns elicited will help you to evaluate impairment (necessary to make the diagnosis) and to identify ongoing treatment goals with the child/young person and family.

Past difficulties

Who first raised concerns? Is the family concerned, or the school, or both? When did the first concerns arise? What were these concerns and how were they handled? Asking about problems experienced in the past is particularly helpful when referral has not taken place until later in childhood (e.g. a 15-year-old adolescent who now 'lounges about' may have been very hyperactive as an 8-year-old child).

Knowing what strategies have been tried in the past, at home and elsewhere (e.g. nursery or school) is helpful for learning about the family's approach and the approach others have taken. Did anything help? Did anything make things worse? Have the family got differing views and styles? Are the family and school currently working together?

Interview with the child/young person

The child/young person, of course, also has an important view, and involving them from the outset is vital. Once the child/young person has met the clinician in their carers' presence, it is good practice to spend time with them alone. When the child is primary-school age it is often better to first conduct information-gathering from them with the carer present, and perhaps at the next appointment to include one-to-one time.

Older children/young people, if invited appropriately, are often keen to share their views, concerns and aspirations. What are their worries, if any? Is there anything they feel they need help with at home or school? How do they feel about friends and peers? They need to be aware of the difficulties being considered and to know how things can be helped. Communication needs to reflect the child/young person's cognitive level, and, if possible, written information designed for their age group should be shared.

Developmental history

The diagnosis of ADHD can only be assessed in the context of that individual's developmental progress. It is beyond the scope of this book to go through typical developmental milestones, but everyone assessing children should already have had experience of developmental assessment. Always ask about progress in gross motor, fine motor, language and social skills. This will help to ascertain the child/young person's developmental level now, their pattern or style of learning, and also point the way to possible additional developmental diagnoses that may either be causing the current symptoms or may be part of comorbid conditions such as general and specific learning difficulties, developmental coordination disorder, language disorder or autism spectrum disorder. If a child/young person has any of these difficulties it does not exclude ADHD – they are in fact at greater risk of the diagnosis – but they do need to be taken into account as they can also mimic ADHD symptoms. The presence of coexisting conditions may also affect management choices (see Chapter 11).

Medical history, including birth history

A thorough medical history is needed to gather information about factors that increase the risk of ADHD and about other difficulties that may cause a symptom profile mimicking ADHD. Some medical issues inform treatment choices and follow-up. Conditions to consider include the following:

• children who were born preterm or who had difficulties around birth

• maternal alcohol or substance misuse in pregnancy

• any brain injury either following trauma or infection (meningitis or encephalitis)

• neurofibromatosis

• tic disorders including Tourette syndrome.

These conditions also increase the individual's risk of having other neurodevelopmental conditions including autism spectrum disorder (ASD), general learning disability and specific learning difficulties.

Epilepsy, particularly absence seizures or some focal epilepsies, may occasionally mimic ADHD but, importantly, there is also an increased incidence of ADHD in individuals who have epilepsy. Children with hearing loss or visual impairment may appear inattentive.

Any significant physical illness may affect a child's well-being, perhaps due to lack of experience of play, frequent hospital admissions or time off school, and this needs to be taken into account when interpreting symptoms.

Medication history

Certain drugs, either prescribed (e.g. anticonvulsants) or when a child/young person is 'self-prescribing' substances, will confuse the presentation and, if ADHD is diagnosed, may affect treatment choices. The use of alcohol, cigarettes and other drugs should be considered and will need ongoing review (see Chapter 15). It may be that a totally truthful response is not forthcoming at the early stages of working with the young person, and parents/carers may be unaware of any substance misuse.

Home environment

Who lives with the child? Are parents together or living separately? Who is the main carer? How many children share the accommodation and the carers? How old are these children and are there any concerns about them? Who else visits? Are the carers in employment? Do the family have financial difficulties? What is the level of education of carers? Have there been any family bereavements? Have there been other disruptions at home (e.g. divorce or domestic abuse)? Are their any housing problems or previous frequent moves? Are their any current or past safeguarding concerns? Is the child adopted? If so what happened prior to the adoption?

Possible attachment disorder may complicate assessment for ADHD and also influence ongoing management. The NICE recommendations (2008) are, however, clear that a child with attachment disorder who fulfils criteria for an ADHD diagnosis should have treatment for ADHD and not only for their attachment disorder.

Family history, including parent/carer physical and mental health

First, as ADHD is a very heritable disorder, ask about symptoms of ADHD in relatives, especially parents and siblings. Go on to enquire about physical problems in the carers that may have impacted parenting. Mental health problems in carers, particularly in the mother, can both impact parenting and be a sign of possible inherited mental health problems in the child. Depression and anxiety are particularly important to consider. If mental health problems are suspected in carers it is helpful to discuss concerns with them and consider referral to their general practitioner (GP) for further assessment and treatment if necessary.

Such information is also important as it may impact the response to management (either behavioural or pharmacological). The presence of untreated parental ADHD significantly worsens the response to behavioural management (Sonuga Barke et al. 2002). Similarly, parental depression or anxiety will affect the parental ability to put in place management strategies (behavioural and medication) and to monitor response.

School life

The school or nursery may have been involved in the referral and you will hopefully have at least some information from them already. Some children seem to manage better at school than at home, but most find school very difficult indeed. You will need information about academic progress and about behaviour in the classroom and during other activities, including play, break times and physical activities.

What strengths does the child have? How does the child/young person feel about school? Have there been frequent changes of school and if so why? Has the child/young person been excluded or truanted? If they are not attending, where are they and with whom? Information about relationships with peers is also relevant. Are there specific concerns about social skills? Is this child/young person involved in bullying or being bullied? Both are more frequent in those with ADHD. Particular teaching styles or subjects can be helpful or otherwise for pupils with ADHD, so ask the child/young person which lessons go better and why they think that is.

Ask parents to bring along any of the child's previous school reports they have. This is particularly useful in children who are not in school, as it can also provide a historical perspective on the child's behaviour as far back as preschool years.

Sleep

Lack of sleep may cause or increase ADHD symptoms. Between 30 and 56% of children/young persons with ADHD have sleep difficulties. This may be difficulty settling to sleep, frequent waking or lack of total sleep time. Families find poor sleep very stressful. Managing a child with ADHD becomes even more difficult when you are sleep-deprived, and a child with ADHD cannot be allowed to be up alone even if they do not disturb everyone. Thinking about sleep at the initial stage is important. Record the average sleep pattern and also ask about snoring and feelings of restlessness in the legs. Discuss bedtime routines. The bedroom environment should be considered. Enquire about any television or computer use before bed. If there are sleep difficulties this is an opportunity to start to put management strategies in place (see Chapter 11).

Coexisting difficulties

There may be additional diagnosed or undiagnosed neurodevelopmental disorders (e.g. learning disability or ASD) or mental health difficulties (e.g. anxiety or depression). Symptoms of any possible coexisting difficulties should be elicited.

Physical examination (Box 3.5)

Physical examination is an important part of the diagnostic process as it may provide clues to other possible diagnoses: either increasing the risk of ADHD, adding to the impairment or mimicking ADHD symptoms. Any additional problems should of course be managed appropriately and the effect on ADHD symptoms assessed.

Dysmorphic features may indicate a chromosomal or other genetic disorder, many of which are linked with learning and sometimes attentional problems. Café-au-lait patches (five or more after age 5) may indicate neurofibromatosis, which requires long-term follow-up. Neurological examination may reveal undiagnosed difficulties.

Box 3.5: Factors to consider in an examination

Physical examination:

✓ Dysmorphism

✓ Neurocutaneous markers

✓ Growth (weight, height, head circumference)

✓ Cardiovascular system (heart sounds, blood pressure, pulse rate)

✓ Neurological examination

Developmental assessment:

✓ Gross motor

✓ Fine motor

✓ Language

✓ Personal/social

Cardiovascular examination is vital as a baseline before considering medication (see Chapter 9). Baseline blood pressure (BP) and pulse rate should be measured. Appendix 2 gives the normal range of blood pressure values taking into account sex, age and height, and Appendix 3 provides normal pulse rate ranges at different ages. This appendix also gives an aide-memoire to correct cuff sizes when measuring BP in childhood. Remember that using too small a cuff will give a falsely high reading.

Very rarely, thyrotoxicosis may mimic ADHD. Consider checking thyroid function if the pulse rate is consistently high at rest or there are any other relevant signs.

Height and weight need to be recorded at baseline and at each visit and plotted on appropriate charts (see Chapter 8). Head circumference should be measured at the initial visit and plotted to look for micro- or macrocephaly, which may need further investigation.

Possible investigation

Investigations are rarely indicated and should be guided by history and examination e.g. chromosomal analysis or microarray if the child has dysmorphic features, and electroencephalogram (EEG) if epilepsy is suspected. Absence epilepsy may masquerade as ADHD (Box 3.6). Careful history, hyperventilation test and EEG will exclude or confirm the diagnosis if it is suspected.

If the child has a history suggestive of restless leg syndrome iron levels should be checked, and if iron deficiency is found, treatment with iron may stop or decrease symptoms.

Box 3.6: Case study

Geraint, aged 8 years

✓ Attended with his mother and stepdad

✓ Concerns raised by school and parents regarding possible ADHD

✓ Finds it difficult to keep attention both at home and school

✓ Is quite forgetful and easily distracted

✓ Finds it difficult to play quietly

✓ Interrupts people

✓ Very impulsive

✓ He was doing well at school but has dropped behind in reading by three levels from September last year

Background

✓ Mother works as a secretary

✓ Parents separated

✓ Some history of learning difficulties on biological dad's side

✓ Lives with his mum, step dad and 3-year-old sibling

✓ There is no other history of ADHD, epilepsy, learning difficulty on mum's side

✓ No neonatal problems

✓ Frequent episodes (3–4 times a week)

✓ Will switch off. No witnessed peri-oral or peri-ocular flickering. No sudden jumps or jerks

✓ School have not noticed these episodes

✓ No significant findings on examination

Hyperventilation test

✓ At around 20 seconds in the test he had an episode during which he became unaware, he was vacantly staring and had some blinking, and parents agreed that this was very similar to the vacant episodes they had noted

✓ Lasted approximately 3-4 seconds

EEG confirmed childhood absence epilepsy treat epilepsy

✓ Responded well to sodium valproate

✓ Still struggles with ADHD symptoms

✓ Then what?

Treat ADHD

✓ Much improved

Observation: clinic, home and school

Observing a child during clinic appointments needs to be interpreted with care (Box 3.7). Even the most affected child can appear to be able to focus and sit quietly for a short period if the situation is right. Sometimes, an apparently very hyperactive child may simply not be used to the situation.

Although full cognitive assessment would be desirable for all children referred for assessment of ADHD, this is not deliverable in current services unless there is a specific indication.

Observation in the structured setting of cognitive testing has, however, been shown to be able to predict the presence or absence of ADHD (e.g. McConaughy et al. 2009). Test examiners used a test observation form to rate behaviour in 6- to 11-year-old children during administration of the Wechsler Intelligence Scale for Children 4th edn (WISC-IV) and Wechsler Individual Achievement Tests 2nd edn (WIAT-II).

Structured school observation

Observation in the paediatric service in Sheffield, UK, is undertaken in school by specialist ADHD nurses or other trained team members (see Chapter 12). They use a structured observation checklist developed by one of the nurses. First, the situation in

---

Box 3.7: Behavioural observation

ADHD may not be observable

✓ In highly structured settings
✓ In novel situations
✓ When patient is engaged in interesting activities
✓ When patient is receiving one-to-one attention
✓ In a controlled and supervised context
✓ Where there are frequent rewards

ADHD typically worsens

✓ In unstructured situations
✓ During repetitive activity
✓ In boring situations
✓ Where there is a lot of distraction
✓ Under minimal supervision
✓ When sustained attention or mental effort is required
✓ During self-paced activities

Observation in varying contexts is important

---

the classroom and the activity/activities being undertaken are noted. The index child/young person is then monitored with respect to a control child recommended by the teacher. Every two minutes for a half-hour period, the observer notes activity levels and symptoms that could represent underlying ADHD. The index child/young person is then scored on a horizontal scale with respect to the whole class.

There is also free text commentary, which would include details of any changes in the environment within the time period and other observations (e.g. symptoms suggestive of ASD or motor difficulties).

The school observation also gives the team access to further information from school. This would include learning levels and, in particular, any known or suspected specific or general learning difficulties. Do teaching staff feel this child/young person is underachieving for their intellectual level? Copies of any educational reports of relevance (test results at various school stages, educational psychology assessments) will be collected (with parental consent). There is also the opportunity to discuss strategies for the classroom. This will be a chance to take into account the current strategies that are being used, to find out what has been helpful and what has not, and to suggest additional strategies if appropriate. Observational visits help to maintain or establish good relationships with individual schools and improve ongoing dialogue and communication. Feedback from school is crucial to the optimisation of treatment.

Additional school information

Some services contact the school by telephone or gain information from teachers using checklists and questionnaires. Team members may have already attended school meetings or had previous contact if the assessment is with a child and family the service already knows for other reasons, but an update is still needed.

In secondary schools, information is needed from several teachers, as teaching style and the type of lesson will affect presentation and the degree of impairment.

Psychological and psychometric assessment

Formal cognitive assessment is neither indicated nor currently available for all children undergoing assessment for possible ADHD. However, educational and clinical psychologists should undertake further assessments if specific learning difficulties, including poor literacy skills, dyslexia or other problems such as dyscalculia or non-verbal learning difficulties, are suspected to be the cause of, or contributing to, attentional difficulties. Any learning issues identified need addressing in their own right.

General learning disabilities may also be present and, if this is suspected, accurate assessment is needed to understand whether any ADHD features are within the average for the child's cognitive level.

Cognitive impairments involving, for example, memory and attention are very likely to be present and ideally should be investigated further by clinical or educational psychologists. In routine clinical practice this is difficult to offer. There are many possible tests. One of the best known is the Test of Everyday Attention for Children (Manly et al. 2001). There are also visual and auditory attentional subtests in neuropsychological batteries that can support or refute the presence of ADHD. The sensitivity and specificity of neuropsychological tests in the diagnosis of ADHD in individual children is poor and, therefore, routine use is not recommended.

Questionnaires

Questionnaires alone cannot diagnose or exclude ADHD. They are, however, extremely important in initial assessment and in monitoring responses to any management undertaken. They also give the opportunity to collect valuable information from multiple sources, including one or more teachers and other carers (e.g. a parent who lives separately but does care for the child at times).

There are also questionnaires for young people themselves. There is evidence showing that self-report is frequently less accurate than the observations of another close individual, but such data are relevant to understanding the young person's point of view and their goals for the future.

Questionnaires can be split into those that consider specific ADHD symptoms only and those that include a broadband assessment of other developmental/mental health difficulties.

ADHD-specific questionnaires usually map to the DSM-IV classification, scoring between 0 (no difference between this child and what would be expected from a child of the same developmental 'age') and 3 (severely affected).

The most commonly questionnaires used in the UK are the Conners Parent Rating Scale (www.mhs.com/conners3) and SNAP-IV (after Swanson, Nolan and Pelham). Both come in short and long forms. The short forms map to ADHD criteria in the DSM-IV, while the long forms gather information around possible differential diagnoses or coexisting difficulties.

The initial Conners Parent Rating Scale was based on 683 children living in Baltimore, USA, in the 1960s, and so the appropriateness of wider application was questioned. A revised version of the scale was published following various studies between 1992 and 1996 and the acquisition of normative data from over 8000 North American children.

The scale uses T scores, which indicate how many standard deviations a particular raw score lies above or below the group mean. In the Conners Rating Scales, 1.5 to 2 standard deviations above the mean indicate a significant problem. Therefore, a raw score that plots a T score above 70 indicates that there is likely to be a significant problem. The long form takes around 20 minutes to complete.

SNAP-IV has a short form looking at ADHD-specific difficulties with 18 questions for parent/carers and for teachers. There is also a longer 80-question form that covers items relating to conduct disorder, Tourette syndrome, stereotypic movement disorder, obsessive-compulsive disorder, generalised anxiety disorder, narcolepsy, histrionic personality disorder, narcissistic personality disorder, borderline personality disorder, manic episode, major depressive episode, dysthymic disorder, post-traumatic stress disorder and adjustment disorder. Finally, the 90-question SNAP-IV includes the 10 items of the Swanson, Kotkin, Agler, Mylnn and Pelham (SKAMP) Rating Scale (Wigal et al. 1998). These items are classroom manifestations of inattention, hyperactivity and impulsivity (i.e. getting started, staying on task, interactions with others, completing work, and shifting activities). The SKAMP (Wigal et al, 1998) may be used to estimate the severity of impairment in the classroom.

Broadband rating scales gather information including scores that describe all types of child behaviour problems, scores that give an indication of depression and anxiety (internalising scale scores) and scores that describe aggression and conduct problems (externalising scale scores). A commonly used example is the Strengths and Difficulties Questionnaire (SDQ; http://www.sdqinfo.org). The SDQ has several different formats, covering different age groups and with or without impact versions. It also has follow-up versions to monitor changes. As its name implies, this does include the collection of information about the child's strengths, which is helpful. Broadband checklist total problem indices or scales assessing externalising, internalising or adaptive behaviour do not screen for or diagnose ADHD. However, they are useful as screening for co-occurring problems in other areas (e.g. anxiety, depression, social skills difficulties or conduct problems). Any high scores in these areas should signpost the need for further relevant assessment.

Questionnaires documenting teachers' views are essential in a diagnostic assessment. If a child/young person is not currently in school, information from previous teachers should be sought. If the child/young person is in a special school, reports from the previous school may be useful too, as a child with ADHD may have significantly less impairment in the small class size and more individual environment of the special school setting. Indeed, ADHD may have caused the behaviours that resulted in the request for special school placement, and effective treatment may negate the need for this placement. In the secondary school, the views of several teachers can be especially useful, indicating types of lessons and styles of teaching that may have a positive or negative effect on the child's impairment. Discussing these with the child and family can be very illuminating.

It is not unusual for parent/carer reporting and teacher reporting to be very different. In a study of the impact of parent and teacher agreement on diagnosing ADHD (Wolraich et al. 2004), inter-rater reliability was low between parent and teacher reports of behaviours. Rates in the sample were similar for parents and teachers in hyperactive/impulsive and combined ADHD, but teacher reports were considerably higher for inattentive symptoms. Discrepancies do not necessarily mean that either report is inaccurate; each rater may be reasonably reliable, but raters observe the child in different situations. Discussion with both reporters can clarify the situation. The DSM criteria require impairment resulting from ADHD behaviours in more than one setting, so resolution of the differences needs to be made.

There are many other questionnaires, including the following:

- *The Vanderbilt Assessment Scale*. This 55-question assessment tool reviews the symptoms of ADHD. It also looks for other conditions such as conduct disorder, oppositional-defiant disorder, anxiety and depression.

- *The Behavior Assessment System for Children (BASC)*. This test looks for things like hyperactivity, aggression and conduct problems. It also looks for anxiety, depression, attention and learning problems, and lack of certain essential skills.

- *The Child Behavior Checklist/Teacher Report Form (CBCL)*. Among other things, this scale looks at physical complaints, aggressive or delinquent behaviour and withdrawal.

It is widely accepted that ADHD adversely affects the quality of life (QoL) of the child/young person and their family (Danckaerts et al. 2010; Peasgood et al. 2016). During assessment, the use of QoL questionnaires is not usual, but this may change if questionnaires which are easy to use in clinical settings become available. This would help to measure and monitor impairment.

Questionnaires that look at function (e.g. the Weiss Functional Impairment Rating Scale (WFIRS), which can be downloaded free from www.caddra.ca) or quality of life (e.g. the Child Health Questionnaire, www.healthact.com) may be helpful to establish a baseline and in monitoring or goal setting.

Bringing it all together

The cornerstone of accurate diagnosis is bringing together carefully collected information from the family, including the child/young person as much as possible, school and other carers. This should build a realistic picture of the child/young person's strengths and their difficulties. These should be considered in terms of practical life events. How does this child interact at home? Is school life difficult and specifically what areas of school life? Can the child/young person join effectively in leisure activities?

Diagnosis is not just about how inattentive, impulsive or hyperactive the child/young person is, but most importantly about how this affects their everyday life. To make a diagnosis of ADHD or attention deficit disorder (ADD) there must be evidence of impairment. The NICE guideline development group found it difficult to define impairment (look back at Box 3.3).

In practice, diagnosis has to be based on a knowledge of what a child/young person of that age and cognitive ability can typically access or do without difficulty or disruption, as well as considering areas in which this child/young person cannot successfully function as expected. This profile informs diagnosis and establishes a baseline on which treatment goals are built to direct and monitor treatment success or otherwise.

Next steps

At this point it may be clear that this child/young person has ADHD or ADD. If so, the management will begin with an explanation of the diagnosis of ADHD and how this diagnosis has been made.

The majority of families whose child is diagnosed with ADHD are relieved to find out that there is an explanation for the difficulties they have experienced and that there is much that can be done to improve things. Sometimes, however, some members of the family may feel the diagnosis is incorrect and feel angry and hostile towards the parent who brought the child for assessment and to the clinician. Time spent explaining the process again, and the reason for the conclusions, is usually well spent, as this is likely to result in increased support for any treatment offered.

During assessment you may have given some information about ADHD to the family. They will often have looked for things themselves. At this point it is appropriate to check what the family already has and to offer additional written information and website addresses. Most teams will have developed a list of good sources of information (Appendix 1 has some I have used). Think about information for the child/young person that is at their developmental level, and do not forget siblings.

A further point which Richard and I find upsetting is Jamie's affect on us as a family, and the effects on our other two boys, aged 10 and 6, who witness temper tantrums, miss out on time with us while we deal/cope with Jamie, hitting them and me. We feel that 75%

of our parenting time and energy are focused on Jamie and the other two suffer for this. They often express that Jamie gets away with naughty behaviour and Adam, our youngest, at times copies him. We have discussed ADHD at age appropriate levels, but they and I find it all difficult to grasp.

(Mother of primary-school-aged boy with ADHD)

Families should also be given details of local parent support groups. They can then decide if and when to contact them. Ongoing care is described in later chapters.

Sometimes it will be clear that the child/young person does not have ADHD or ADD. If this is the case, any possible comorbid difficulties should be explored and, if necessary, further assessment of these should be planned. If no developmental or mental health difficulty is suspected, the child/young person and family should be signposted to other support and discharged.

However, the diagnosis is not always clear after thorough initial assessment. Sometimes a decision may be made to wait. For example, if a child is seen in the summer holidays it may be helpful to review the situation when they have settled into the new class, or, if there are specific difficulties at home that make interpretation of symptoms impossible, then support should be given prior to review.

If the assessment has revealed the likelihood of other developmental or mental health conditions or medical problems that may mimic or mask ADHD, these should be assessed further and treatment and support put in place. If these are felt to cause the full difficulties and ADHD is felt to have been excluded, follow-up will be with other relevant services. Chapter 4 discusses assessment for coexisting conditions further, and Chapter 11 the effect these may have on management.

Computerised tests

Another possible addition to diagnostic assessment is the use of computer tests. One example we have used is the Quantified Behaviour Test (Qb test; see https://www.qbtech.com), which involves the child/young person doing a test, where they have to respond differently depending on the image displayed (e.g. red or blue square or triangle). The child wears a headband with a marker on it and this is used to detect their pattern of movement during the test. The number of correct responses, incorrect responses, omitted responses and variability are compared with normal values. The test takes around 30 minutes to administer, including test instructions. The test pattern may also suggest learning difficulties or ASD. Several other systems are also effective. These include the Test of Variables of Attention (T.O.V.A, The TOVA Company, www.tovatest.com), which measures key components of attention and self control, variability (consistency), response time (speed), commissions (impulsivity) and omissions (focus and vigilance), the Conners Continuous Performance Test, 3rd edn, which measures performance in areas of inattentiveness, impulsivity, sustained attention and vigilance (www.MHS.com), and a number of tests from Cambridge Cognition (www.cambridgecognition.com).

None of these provides a single test for ADHD, but they are increasingly supporting full clinical assessment.

Summary

- Diagnostic assessment teams vary greatly across the UK, Europe and worldwide.

- Each team needs all the relevant competencies.

- Diagnosing ADHD needs a careful structured approach.

- Information from multiple sources is always required.

- Functional impairment caused by ADHD symptoms must be assessed and recorded.

- Comorbid conditions must be considered.

- A step-by-step approach is most successful in achieving timely and accurate diagnosis.

References

American Psychiatric Association (2013) *Diagnostic and statistical manual of mental disorders*, 5th edn. Arlington, VA: American Psychiatric Association.

Behavior Assessment System for Children; available at www.pearsonclinical.co.uk.

Child Behavior Checklist/Teacher Report Form; available at www.aseba.org.

Danckaerts M, Sonuga Barke E, Banaschewski T et al. (2010) The quality of life of children with attention deficit/hyperactivity disorder: A systematic review. *Eur Child Adolesc Psychiatry* 19(2): 83–105.

Manly T, Nimmo-Smith I, Watson P, Anderson V, Turner A, Robertson I (2001) The differential assessment of children's attention: The Test of Everyday Attention for Children (TEA-Ch), normative sample and ADHD performance. *J Child Psychol Psychiatry* 42: 1065–1081.

McConaughy S, Ivanova M, Antshel K, Eiraldi R (2009) Standardized observational assessment of attention deficit hyperactivity disorder combined and predominantly inattentive subtypes. I. Test session observations. *School Psych Rev* 38(1): 45–66.

NICE (2008) *Attention deficit hyperactivity disorder: Diagnosis and management. NICE Clinical Guidelines* [CG72], https://www.nice.org.uk/guidance/cg72.

Peasgood T, Bhardwaj A, Biggs K et al. (2016) The impact of ADHD on the health and well-being of ADHD children and their siblings. *Eur Child Adolesc Psychiatry* 2016, doi:10.1007/s00787-016-0841-6.

Shaw M, Hodgkins P, Caci H et al. (2012) A systematic review and analysis of long-term outcomes in attention deficit hyperactivity disorder: Effects of treatment and non-treatment. *BMC Med* 10: 99.

Sonuga-Barke EJ, Daley D, Thompson M (2002) Does maternal ADHD reduce the effectiveness of parent training for preschool children's ADHD? *J Am Acad Child Adolesc Psychiatry* 41: 696–702.

Vanderbilt Assessment Scale; available at www.nichq.org/childrens-health/adhd/resources/vanderbilt-assessment-scales).

Wigal SB, Gupta S, Guinta D, Swanson JM (1998) Reliability and validity of the SKAMP rating scale in a laboratory school setting. *Psychopharmacol Bull* 34: 47–53.

Wolraich ML, Lambert EW, Bickman L, Simmons T, Doffing MA, Worley KA (2004) Assessing the impact of parent and teacher agreement on diagnosing attention-deficit hyperactivity disorder. *J Dev Behav Paediatr* 25(1): 41–47.

Chapter 4

Coexisting difficulties

Val Harpin

This chapter will consider other neurodevelopmental and mental health disorders that commonly coexist with ADHD and which may also complicate assessment. We will think about tools to help in the diagnosis of these disorders and signs that indicate the need for further assessment. In Chapter 11 we will explore how comorbid conditions may affect treatment choice and success.

The presence of comorbid conditions has been shown to adversely affect quality of life for children and young people with ADHD and their families (Klassen et al. 2004; Newcorn et al. 2005). It is therefore vital to recognise any comorbid conditions and adjust management appropriately to optimise outcomes.

Prevalence

It is difficult to be precise about the prevalence of comorbid conditions, as reports differ widely due to the clinical, research or community populations they examine. In each case the range from different studies is given. Perhaps the best information for some comorbid conditions comes from a total-population-based study in Sweden. It showed that 87% of children meeting full criteria for ADHD using DSM-III-R (3.7% of the population) had one or more comorbidities and 67% had at least two comorbid diagnoses. The most common comorbidities were oppositional defiant disorder (60%) and developmental coordination disorder (47%) This study also reports a 7% incidence of Asperger syndrome, despite the fact that at that time pervasive developmental disorder was considered to exclude the diagnosis of ADHD (Kadesjö & Gillberg 2001).

The Multimodal Treatment of Attention Deficit Hyperactivity Disorder (MTA) study included a study group of 600 children and young people with ADHD (MTA Cooperative Group 1999). This reported the following prevalences of comorbid conditions:

- 33.5% anxiety disorder

- 14.3% conduct disorder

- 39.9% oppositional defiant disorder

- 3.8% affective disorder

- 10.9% tic disorder

- 31.8% no comorbid condition

However, the prevalence of comorbidity in this study is less generalisable to current clinical practice, as it did not investigate some major comorbidities.

Full definitions of the comorbid mental health and neurodevelopmental disorders can be found either in DSM-5 (American Psychiatric Association 2013) or the International Statistical Classification of Diseases and Related Health Problems, 10th revision (ICD-10, WHO, n.d.).

Oppositional defiant disorder

Oppositional defiant disorder (ODD) is reported to be present in between 40 and 80% of children and young people with ADHD. It is defined within the grouping Disruptive, Impulse-Control, and Conduct Disorders in DSM-5. ODD usually occurs in younger children and is primarily characterised by markedly defiant, disobedient, and disruptive behaviour that does not include delinquent acts or the more extreme forms of aggressive or dissocial behaviour (see section 'Conduct disorder').

Severely mischievous or naughty behaviour does not itself qualify for the diagnosis. DSM-5 describes ODD as a pattern of angry/irritable mood and argumentative/defiant behaviour, or vindictiveness as evidenced by at least four symptoms from a list of behaviours in the above two categories.

The behaviours must have been present for at least 6 months and must occur during interaction with at least one individual who is not a sibling. As normal childhood behaviour can include such behaviours, the persistence and frequency should be used to distinguish a behaviour that is within normal limits from a behaviour that is diagnostic.

DSM-5 defines this as follows:

- for children younger than 5 years, behaviour occurring on most days for a period of at least 6 months;

- for individuals 5 years or older, behaviour occurring at least once per week for at least 6 months.

Other factors should also be considered, such as whether the frequency and intensity of the behaviours are outside the expected range for the individual's developmental level, sex and culture.

The behaviour must be associated with distress in the individual or others in his or her immediate social context (e.g. family, peer group, work colleagues) and must affect social, educational, occupational or other important areas of functioning.

The definition also excludes other causes of such behaviour (e.g. a psychotic episode, substance misuse, depressive or bipolar disorder).

It is likely that having ADHD contributes to and in some cases causes ODD in these individuals, particularly if untreated or diagnosed late. If a child or young person has both ADHD and ODD, the symptoms of ADHD always pre-date ODD. It is perhaps understandable that a young child who is constantly being told off, usually without understanding why, begins to behave less well. At least some ODD is related to a disrupted parenting style, and when at least one parent has ADHD themselves the risk of ODD is four times higher. The presence of ODD predicts the persistence of ADHD symptoms.

Effective management of ADHD before a child has ODD symptoms may be instrumental in avoiding progression to ODD, although there is currently no evidence to prove this. Support for preschool children with ADHD and their families is likely to be particularly helpful if the parent/child relationship can be improved and ADHD symptoms understood and improved at an early age.

Conduct disorder

Conduct disorder is reported to coexist with ADHD in 20–56% of children and young people. Again, this large variation results from differences between the populations assessed.

Conduct disorder is diagnosed when a child or young person exhibits a repetitive and persistent pattern of behaviour in which the basic rights of others or major age-appropriate societal norms or rules are violated.

Box 4.1: Conduct disorder

Categories considered in diagnosis (DSM-5):

✓ Aggression to people and animals

✓ Destruction of property

✓ Deceitfulness or theft

✓ Serious violations of rules

DSM-5 further defines conduct disorder using four categories of behaviour (Box 4.1) and lists a total of 15 examples of these behaviours. Some behaviours must have been present for the last 12 months.

Conduct disorder can usefully be considered in two groups: early onset and later onset.

Group 1 – Early onset

This group have the following characteristics:

• usually show more severe and more persistent antisocial behaviour

• associated with worse family psychopathology

• often less responsive to treatment

• likely to have a significant genetic component

Group 2 – Later onset (>12 years)

This group has the following characteristics:

• more commonly related to social disadvantage

• associated with increased family disruption, divorce or absent fathers

• major depression more likely to coexist in the child/young person and family members

• school dropout, poor peer group and teen pregnancy risk increased

Anxiety disorders

Significant anxiety disorder is reported in 10–40% of individuals with ADHD. An anxiety disorder is differentiated from the typical fears or anxieties of childhood by being excessive, unusual for the situation or persisting beyond developmentally appropriate time periods. Anxiety must be experienced more days than not for more than 6 months.

The child/young person must have significant difficulty controlling the anxieties and must exhibit one or more of the following: restlessness, fatigue, poor concentration, irritability, muscle tension and sleep disturbance. Several of these are seen in ADHD, but the causation must be clearly anxiety to merit the second diagnosis and, once again, symptoms must not be explainable by other diagnoses.

Comorbid anxiety disorder is seen more frequently

- in girls

- when there is also coexisting autism spectrum disorder (ASD)

- in association with poor emotional regulation

- when there is a family history of anxiety disorder

In all assessments, interviewing the child/young person alone is important in order to obtain a report of symptoms or difficulties first hand, but it is particularly so when an anxiety disorder is suspected. It is helpful to explore the young person's underlying thoughts and fears. It is also important to elicit symptoms and difficulties that may not have been shared with the carer. Anxiety can often present as a consequence of untreated moderate to severe ADHD, so early diagnosis of ADHD and optimal management of ADHD symptoms are imperative and improve the prognosis in those who have coexisting anxiety.

Depression

Depression is significantly more common in children and young people with ADHD than in those without ADHD. However, the reported prevalence of depression in individuals with ADHD once again varies greatly in different community or clinical cohorts (between 0 and 45%). Depression affects females more than males, commonly presents in older children, and again is more likely to be associated with those who have ADHD that has been missed or not optimally managed. Those affected, particularly females, commonly internalise their difficulties, leading to depression.

The depressive disorders are defined in full in DSM-5. The common feature of these disorders is the presence of low mood, with a loss of enjoyment in previously pleasurable activities (anhedonia). Low mood can present as sadness, irritability or even anger in young people. These features are accompanied by somatic and cognitive changes that significantly affect the individual's capacity to function.

Studies suggest a moderate genetic linkage between ADHD and depression (Cross-Disorder Group of the Psychiatric Genomics Consortium 2013), and the risk of depression is also increased by the presence of conduct disorder in the child or a family member.

Depression may be manifest as low self-esteem in childhood, and full onset may not occur until adolescence or later. Humphreys et al. (2013) used two cohorts, one of children aged 5–10 years and one follow-up study from birth to 20 years, to investigate mediators of depression in individuals with ADHD. Both studies implicated peer and parent–child problems as unique mediators of depressive symptoms. Inattention symptoms, but not hyperactivity, also predicted depressive symptoms.

Individuals with ADHD and comorbid depression have increased risk of suicidal ideation and attempts. Chronis-Tuscano and colleagues (2010) found that children with ADHD diagnosed at 4–6 years of age were at greatly increased risk for meeting DSM-IV criteria for major depression or dysthymia (hazard ratio, 4.32) and for attempting suicide (hazard ratio, 3.60) through to the age of 18 years relative to comparison children. Within the ADHD group, girls were at greater risk for depression and suicide attempts. Maternal depression and concurrent child emotional and behavioural problems at 4–6 years of age also predicted depression and suicidal behaviour.

Sleep disorders

Between 30 and 56% of children diagnosed with ADHD have disordered sleep at the time of diagnosis. This is principally delayed onset, and more frequent night wakenings leading to shorter sleep time. Families also report more activity during sleep.

Disordered sleep may exacerbate and even cause ADHD-like symptoms. It is vital therefore to take a detailed history of any reported sleep problems at the time of assessment and to institute strategies to improve sleep (see Chapter 11). Organic causes of disordered sleep such as sleep apnoea and restless legs syndrome should be considered and investigated further if symptoms suggest their presence. During the treatment of ADHD, medication may worsen sleep difficulties.

Neurodevelopmental disorders

Under the heading Neurodevelopmental Disorders, DSM-5 lists the following:

- intellectual disability
- communication disorders
- autism spectrum disorder (ASD)

- ADHD

- specific learning disorder

- motor disorders

- developmental coordination disorder

- tics and Tourette syndrome

- stereotyped movements

These disorders are characterised by onset in the early developmental period, skills below those expected for chronological age and significant impairment of function.

Other causes for the symptoms must also have been excluded. Some of these difficulties will be considered independently, but, as clinicians are becoming more aware of the complexity of neurodevelopmental profiles, it has become very clear that children and young people often do not fit into neat diagnostic boxes. Many individuals have traits of different neurodevelopmental disorders, although they may not fulfil the full criteria for all, if any, diagnoses. Such individuals may have been born preterm or have suffered some brain injury. The assessment of ADHD is then especially challenging but particularly important as treatment, although often also more challenging, can be extremely positive for the quality of life of both the child and family.

Intellectual disability/general learning disability

The prevalence of ADHD in individuals with general learning disability is unknown, but studies suggest that it is between 18 and 40% (Pliszka 2015). In the past, ADHD symptoms have often been attributed to the learning disability, but clinicians are increasingly assessing, diagnosing and treating individuals in this vulnerable group.

Clearly, the key challenge is to assess ADHD in line with the child/young person's cognitive/developmental ability and ascertain whether there is a mismatch between the two. Thus, professionals undertaking clinical evaluation should have expertise in both ADHD and learning disability, and awareness of the normal range of behaviour in the equivalent peer group of comparable age and general cognitive ability. Education staff, and in particular special needs teachers and educational psychologists, can be extremely helpful in making this judgement.

ADHD has been particularly underdiagnosed in this group, but it has become increasingly clear that treatment can be extremely useful (Simonoff et al. 2013) and that treatment can improve the quality of life of the individual and their carers.

Communication disorders

Young children with ADHD often have delayed but not disordered language, possibly secondary to poor listening skills and lack of participation in language use. However, all types of communication disorder are also more common and, if there is concern, referral to a speech and language therapist is indicated to ensure that appropriate assessment and treatment is offered.

Communication disorders fall into five categories:

- receptive and expressive language disorders

- speech sound disorders

- childhood onset fluency disorder

- social (pragmatic) communication disorder

- unspecified communication disorder

In this context, only social communication disorder is considered further.

Autism spectrum disorder

The prevalence of ASD in the general population is known to be around 1%, substantially greater than previously recognised (Baird et al. 2006). Whether the increase is due to better ascertainment, broadening diagnostic criteria or increased incidence is unclear.

DSM-IV precluded a double diagnosis of ADHD and pervasive developmental disorder. As a result, the prevalence of diagnostic overlap is not fully understood. Overlap on a symptom level is very common in clinical practice. Clark et al. (1999) studied autistic features in children and young people with ADHD using the parent-rated Autism Criteria Checklist. A high proportion of parents (between 65 and 80%) reported significant difficulties in social interaction (particularly in empathy and peer relationships) and communication (particularly in imaginative ability, non-verbal communication and maintaining conversation). Also, clinicians were aware of many individuals in whom a diagnosis of ASD was preceded by a diagnosis of ADHD and unmasked by treatment to reduce ADHD symptoms.

The NICE Guideline (2008) recognised the coexistence of ASD and ADHD, and DSM-5 also now describes their coexistence.

DSM-5 reviewed the diagnostic criteria for ASD. A single category of ASD is now used that subsumes previous subtypes, including Asperger syndrome and high functioning autism. Clinicians are now expected to develop a matrix that describes the strengths and difficulties of this particular individual with ASD. Such a matrix should describe the severity of each component, the course of the disorder (e.g. any skill loss, intellectual ability, language competence and any additional physical or mental health difficulties). Using such a matrix can be extremely helpful to map progress and to share information with schools. Each individual with ASD has a unique profile. Being aware that 'one size' does not fit all needs is vital to optimising support. In the context of ADHD, changes in ADHD symptoms and how they interact with ASD symptoms can be monitored using the matrix format and specific symptom questionnaires.

In DSM-5, the triad of impairments previously used in the assessment of ASD has been reduced to a dyad:

- persistent deficits in social communication and social understanding across multiple contexts, either current or by history (Box 4.2)

- restricted, repetitive patterns of behaviour, interests or activities, currently or by history (Box 4.3)

Some features of each area in Box 4.2 (social skills) and two of the four in Box 4.3 must be present currently or in the history to make the diagnosis.

As with other neurodevelopmental disorders, symptoms must be present in the early developmental period, cause clinically significant impairment in social, occupational or other areas of current functioning, and cannot be better explained by other diagnoses.

Box 4.2: Autism spectrum disorder (A)

A. Persistent deficits in social communication and social interaction across multiple contexts:

✓ Deficits in social-emotional reciprocity
  - Abnormal social approach and failure of normal back-and-forth conversation
  - Reduced sharing of interests, emotions or affect
  - Failure to initiate or respond to social interactions
✓ Deficits in non-verbal communicative behaviours used for social interaction
  - Poorly integrated verbal and non-verbal communication
  - Abnormalities in eye contact and body language and deficits in understanding and use of gestures
  - Total lack of facial expressions and non-verbal communication
✓ Deficits in developing, maintaining and understanding relationships
  - Difficulties in adjusting behaviour to suit various social contexts
  - Difficulties in sharing imaginative play or in making friends
  - Absence of interest in peers

Box 4.3: Autism spectrum disorder (B)

B. Restricted, repetitive patterns of behaviour, interests or activities:

✓ Stereotyped or repetitive motor movements, use of objects or speech:
- Simple motor stereotypes
- Lining up toys or flipping objects
- Echolalia
- Idiosyncratic phrases

✓ Insistence on sameness, inflexible adherence to routines or ritualised patterns of verbal or non-verbal behaviour:
- Extreme distress at small changes
- Difficulties with transitions
- Rigid thinking patterns
- Greeting rituals
- Need to take same route or eat the same food every day

✓ Highly restricted, fixated interests that are abnormal in intensity or focus:
- Strong attachment to or preoccupation with unusual objects
- Excessively circumscribed or perseverative interests

✓ Hyper- or hyporeactivity to sensory input or unusual interest in sensory aspects of the environment:
- Apparent indifference to pain/temperature
- Adverse response to specific sounds or textures
- Excessive smelling or touching of objects
- Visual fascination with lights or movement

Social communication disorder

The term 'social communication disorder' is especially useful in describing the difficulties some children and young people with ADHD have with social communication (Box 4.4). This includes some characteristics of the social communication difficulties seen in ASD in an individual without restricted interests or rigidity.

Such difficulties are particularly evident and impairing in secondary-school-age groups when language becomes more abstract and peer relationships more complex. When linked with impulsivity and lack of focus, major issues can arise with peers and with teachers.

Box 4.4: Social (pragmatic) communication disorder

Persistent difficulties in the social use of verbal and non-verbal communication as manifested by all of the following:

✓ Deficits in using communication for social purposes, such as greetings and sharing information, in a manner that is appropriate for the social context

✓ Impairment of the ability to change communication to match context or the needs of the listener, such as speaking differently in a classroom from in a playground, talking differently to a child than to an adult, and avoiding the use of overly formal language

✓ Difficulties following the rules for conversation and story-telling, such as taking turns in a conversation, rephrasing when misunderstood, and knowing how to use verbal and non-verbal signals to regulate interaction

✓ Difficulties understanding what is not explicitly stated (e.g. making inferences) and non-literal or ambiguous meanings of language (e.g. idioms, humour, metaphors, multiple meanings that depend on context for interpretation)

Specific learning difficulties

Specific learning difficulties (SpLD) should be considered where children/young people struggle with literacy or numeracy to a degree that would not be expected for a child of their general ability.

Formal diagnosis of SpLD is usually made by education-based professionals such as specialist teachers or educational psychologists, but clinicians assessing for ADHD must consider their presence as they can mimic ADHD symptoms.

Children who have otherwise good cognitive ability are often aware of specific literacy or mathematical difficulties and may avoid having their problems shown up by becoming the class clown. Children who cannot read or write well will often daydream in classroom situations as they cannot progress. Assessment for SpLD may not be easily available and some families arrange private assessments. Recognition is important, however, as specific teaching methods can be very helpful and may avoid incorrect diagnosis of ADHD.

Developmental coordination disorder

Between 20 and 50% of individuals with ADHD have coexisting developmental coordination disorder (DCD). It is, however, frequently undiagnosed in children and young people with ADHD. Parents may bring concerns to the clinician, or teachers may notice significant motor difficulties in school. The criteria for the diagnosis of DCD are described in Box 4.5.

> **Box 4.5:** Developmental coordination disorder
>
> To meet the criteria for diagnosis of DCD, an individual must demonstrate motor performance that
>
> ✓ is substantially below expected levels given the child's chronological age and appropriate opportunities for skill acquisition
>
> ✓ significantly interferes with activities of daily living or academic achievement
>
> ✓ is not solely explainable by learning disability
>
> ✓ cannot be explained by any specific congenital or acquired neurological disorder, e.g. mild cerebral palsy or any severe psychosocial problem

Usually, diagnosis is made by joint assessment by a paediatrician and either a physio-therapist or an occupational therapist. Physical examination must be undertaken to exclude other possible causes of motor difficulty, and further assessment with a specific test for DCD such as the Movement ABC is needed to demonstrate the level of difficulty. The European Academy of Childhood Disability (EACD) produced detailed guidelines on the assessment and treatment of DCD in 2011 (http://www.eacd. org/publications.php).

Tic disorders

Between 10 and 15% of children and young people with ADHD also have significant tics. A tic is a sudden, rapid, recurrent, involuntary stereotyped motor movement or vocalisation.

Motor tics include blinking, grimacing and head/neck/shoulder movements, and examples of vocal tics include coughing, throat clearing and repeating words or phrases. Tics are typically worsened by anxiety or boredom and by being asked or expected to stop.

Tourette syndrome

Tourette syndrome is named after the French doctor, Georges Gilles de la Tourette, who first described the syndrome and its symptoms in the 19th century. To be diag-nosed with Tourette syndrome the individual must have both multiple motor and one or more vocal tics present for more than a year.

Around 10% of individuals with Tourette syndrome display coprolalia (excessive/ inappropriate swearing), and this is not an essential part of the diagnosis. In most individuals with ADHD, excessive swearing is more likely to be due to excessive exposure to swearing than to Tourette syndrome, but clearly a history of other tics should always be sought. Tourette syndrome occurs in fewer than 2% of individuals with ADHD, but ADHD occurs in 50–80% of those with Tourette syndrome. Great Ormond Street Hospital in London has produced a number of helpful leaflets on Tourette syndrome, including leaflets for parents, young people and teachers, and including a specific section on Tourette syndrome and ADHD. These can be accessed at http://www.gosh.nhs.uk/medical-information/ search-medical-conditions/tourette-syndrome/tourette-syndrome- information-pack.

Epilepsy and ADHD

ADHD is common in children with epilepsy (three to five times the prevalence in the general population). ADHD usually pre-dates seizures (Herman et al. 2007). Davis et al. (2010) reviewed the medical records of children with and without ADHD up to the age of 20 years, and found that those with ADHD were 2.7 times more likely to have epilepsy than those without. Epilepsy in children with ADHD appeared to be more severe than in those without, and there appeared to be a reluctance to diagnose and initiate treatment for ADHD in children with epilepsy.

Electroencephalogram (EEG) abnormality is also common in ADHD (19% in a study of 42 children with ADHD; Sylvestri et al. 2007), but this is not diagnostic of epilepsy and should be interpreted with caution. Further research is needed about the relevance of abnormality in sleep EEG, particularly in children with language disorders or DCD as comorbidity. Diagnosing epilepsy hinges on very careful history taking, not EEG findings. If episodes that may be seizures are reported, recording a video on a mobile phone can be very useful.

As described in Chapter 3, differential diagnosis can be difficult when considering ADHD, and occasionally children with absence epilepsy or complex partial seizures may present with 'attentional difficulties'. A child or young person who is known to have epilepsy has additional possible causative factors for cognitive and behavioural difficulties that must be considered. These include the underlying disease state that causes the epilepsy and the psychosocial disruption in their lifestyles that seizures may produce. Antiepileptic drugs (AEDs) may also affect attention, cognitive ability and behaviour (Anderson et al. 2015). Drane and Meador provide an excellent overview of the cognitive and behavioural effects of AEDs (Drane & Meador 2002). It is important, however, that clinicians do not assume that medication is at fault and fail to consider coexisting ADHD. There has been concern about possible seizure-promoting effects from some medications used in the treatment of ADHD, but the evidence is now considered to be poor (Feldman et al 1989; Gross-Tsur et al. 1997).

Reactive attachment disorder

The concept of attachment disorder was developed by Bowlby (1982) and has been further refined since. Children with reactive attachment disorder, as described in DSM-5, may show social disinhibition, but not the full ADHD symptom cluster, and display other features (such as a lack of enduring relationships) that are not characteristic of

ADHD. It is not uncommon, however, to find that children being seen for the assessment of possible ADHD have in their past histories features that may raise concerns about attachment disorder. It is important to consider this carefully and not jump to conclusions. Some children and young people display great resilience to adversity, and others are deeply affected. Appropriate support should be offered to explore ongoing needs. If the child/young person fulfils criteria for ADHD, this diagnosis should be made, treatment should be given. Families, natural or adoptive, should not be denied treatment for ADHD while treatment for possible attachment is awaited. For more detail about reactive attachment disorder, see Hanson and Spratt (2000).

Developing a toolkit to investigate coexisting conditions

A great deal of information about possible coexisting disorders will be gleaned from detailed history-taking, but during an ADHD assessment, many additional clues may be apparent, and looking for these should be built into the assessment at every opportunity.

Every assessing clinician needs to develop a toolkit to help them to identify likely comorbid conditions. Broadband questionnaires may also be helpful, and both will signpost the need for further assessment or referral to others who can do this.

First impressions when the child/young person comes into the room
- *Eye contact:* Is this given or withheld? What is the quality of eye contact?

- *Greeting:* Does the child/young person greet you appropriately on arrival? Are they over friendly or aloof?

- *Facial expression:* Do they look sad? Anxious? Disinterested? Angry?

- *Posture:* Look at their style of walking in or sitting; e.g. sliding off the chair may suggest motor control problems?

- *Clothing/image:* Are they dressed appropriately for their age and situation?

Behaviour in clinic and in and out of school
Clearly, the assessment includes information about behaviours relevant to ADHD. In addition you should include information about friendships and social interaction with family members, peers and others (e.g. teachers in various settings).

Mood: Look for evidence of low mood, anxiety, mania and excessive mood swings.

Tics (motor and vocal): these should be documented. Remember they are likely to be more frequent if the child/young person is anxious or bored.

Language and communication

Think about the areas described in the following as you engage in conversation with the child/young person. Consciously discussing areas of interest to them, attempting to share humour, a book or play can be extremely valuable.

- *Language complexity:* Is their language too simple for their age, suggesting learning or language difficulties, or does it sound too 'grown up', perhaps suggesting ASD?

- *Conversation/language:* Does the child/young person have an interest in limited topics and show little awareness of others' interest or lack of it?

- *Reciprocal/interest in others:* Do they join in with conversations of interest to others and welcome comments and views from others in their own choice of conversation?

- *Humour:* Do they 'get' humour at an age-appropriate level?

- *Literality of interpretation:* Does literal interpretation of language cause misunderstanding and problems? Is understanding tone of voice and facial expression difficult? You can try out a few simple tests in clinic:

  - 'Pull yourself together'

  - 'Raining cats and dogs'

  - 'I'm going to lose my rag with you!'

  - 'You can go swimming when this glass is empty'

  - 'That's a bit of a kick in the teeth'

  - 'Yeah. Course I'll go out with you'

Obsessional traits

They should be specifically asked about both current and past behaviour. Collecting popular items is common at some ages, but collections of unusual intensity or unusual items (e.g. paperclips, stones) may be related to ASD.

Simple screens for motor problems

In the assessment room, using a pegboard or plastic nut and bolt will help demonstrate difficulties with dexterity. Spotty dogs (when standing, moving the arm and leg on the same side together repetitively) is fun and easy to get young people to try. Asking the child to sit on the floor and get up, first of all as quickly as they can and then without putting hands down can demonstrate coordination difficulties. The Fogg Test is also a simple screen. Ask the child to walk on heels and outside and inside of their feet and look for asymmetry and associated movements of upper limbs and tongue.

Writing is often an additional impairment in school, and getting the child/young person to write in their notes is usually popular and can be referred back to after treatment.

Note difficulties with spelling and in older children letter reversal, which may indicate the need for further assessment for SpLD.

Investigations

Investigations are not indicated in pure ADHD, but the need will be influenced by the presence of any associated conditions. A hearing test is essential if there is any query about hearing, and vision testing may also be indicated if inattention is particularly seen in some school activities. In those with general learning disability, karyotype or microarray analysis should be considered and is essential if there are any dysmorphic features on examination. Imaging (brain magnetic resonance imaging (MRI) or computed tomography (CT)) may be appropriate if a child has an unusually large or small head circumference or if they have more than five café au lait patches or any unusual depigmented skin patches (possible neurofibromatosis or tuberose sclerosis).

EEG is only indicated if there is a suspicion of epilepsy to help define seizure type. Electrocardiogram and echocardiogram may be needed to investigate a possible cardiac anomaly or if there is relevant family history (see Chapter 9) but not as a routine.

Summary

- Every child/young person deserves a holistic assessment and a full description of their areas of need. Only then can a full package of support be put in place. Often impairments in different areas can be reduced by specific support and this will contribute to overall improvement in well-being and quality of life.

- Consider referrals to others in the core team and to those in wider health services (e.g. speech and language therapist, psychologist, physiotherapist, occupational therapist, neurologist) and beyond to other agencies. In particular, liaising with education about all areas of difficulty will optimise support in school.

- In Chapter 11 we will look further at available management strategies for coexisting difficulties.

References

American Psychiatric Association (2013) *Diagnostic and statistical manual of mental disorders*, 5th edn. Arlington, VA: American Psychiatric Association.

Anderson M, Egunsola O, Cherrill J, Millward C, Fakis A, Choonara I (2015) A prospective study of adverse drug reactions to antiepileptic drugs in children. *Br Med J* 5(6): e008298, doi: 10.1136/bmjopen-2015-008298.

Baird G, Simonoff E, Pickles A et al. (2006) Prevalence of disorders of the autism spectrum in a population cohort of children in South Thames: the Special Needs and Autism Project (SNAP). *Lancet* 368(9531): 210–215, doi:10.1016/S0140-6736(06)69041-7.

Bowlby J (1982) Attachment and loss: Attachment. In: *Attachment and loss*, Vol. 1, Basic Books Classics, Issue 79 of International Psycho-analytical Library. New York, NY: Basic Books.

Clark T, Feehan C, Tinline C, Vostanis P (1999) Autistic symptoms in children with attention deficit–hyperactivity disorder. *Eur Child Adolesc Psychiatry* 8: 50–55, doi:10.1007/s007870050083.

Chronis-Tuscano A, Molina BSG, Pelham WE et al. (2010) Very early predictors of adolescent depression and suicide attempts in children with attention-deficit/hyperactivity disorder. *Arch Gen Psychiatry* 67(10): 1044–1051, doi:10.1001/archgenpsychiatry.2010.127.

Cross-Disorder Group of the Psychiatric Genomics Consortium (2013) Genetic relationship between five psychiatric disorders estimated from genome-wide SNPs. *Nat Genet* 45(9): 984–994, doi:10.1038/ng.2711.

Davis SM, Katusic SK, Barbaresi WJ et al. (2010) Epilepsy in children with ADHD: A population-based study. *Pediatr Neurol* 42(5): 325–330, doi: 10.1016/j.pediatrneurol.2010.01.005.

Drane D, Meador K (2002) Cognitive and behavioral effects of antiepileptic drugs. *Epilepsy Behav* 3: S49–S53.

Feldman H, Cumrine P, Handen BL et al. (1989) Methylphenidate in children with seizures and attention-deficit disorder. *Am J Dis Child* 143: 1081–1086.

Gross-Tsur V, Manor O, van der Meere J et al. (1997) Epilepsy and attention deficit hyperactivity disorder: Is methylphenidate safe and effective? *J Pediatrics* 130: 40–44.

Hanson R, Spratt E (2000) Reactive attachment disorder: What we know about the disorder and implications for treatment. *Child Maltreat* 5(2): 137–145, doi:10.1177/1077559500005002005.

Herman B, Jones J, Dabbs K et al. (2007) The frequency, complications and aetiology of ADHD in new onset paediatric epilepsy. *Brain* 130: 3135–3148, doi:10.1093/brain/awm227 3135-3148.

Humphreys KL, Katz SJ, Lee SS, Hammen CL, Brennan PA, Najman JM (2013) The association of ADHD and depression: Mediation by peer problems and parent–child difficulties in two complementary samples. *J Abnorm Psychol* 122(3): 854–867, doi:10.1037/a0033895.

Kadesjö B, Gillberg C (2001) The comorbidity of ADHD in the general population of Swedish school-age children. *J Child Psychol Psychiatry* 42(4): 487–492, doi:10.1111/1469-7610.00742.

Klassen AF, Miller A, Fine S (2004) Health-related quality of life in children and adolescents who have a diagnosis of attention-deficit/hyperactivity disorder. *Pediatrics* 114(5): e541, doi:10.1542/peds.2004-0844.

MTA Cooperative Group (1999) A 14-month randomized clinical trial of treatment strategies for attention-deficit/hyperactivity disorder (ADHD). *Arch Gen Psychiatry* 56: 1073–1086.

Movement Assessment Battery for Children; available at http://www.pearsonclinical.co.uk/Psychology/ ChildCognitionNeuropsychologyandLanguage/ChildPerceptionandVisuomotorAbilities/ MABC-2/MovementAssessmentBatteryforChildren-SecondEdition(MovementABC-2).aspx.

Newcorn J, Spencer T, Biederman J, Milton D, Michelson D (2005) Atomoxetine treatment in children and adolescents with attention-deficit/hyperactivity disorder and comorbid oppositional defiant disorder. *J Am Acad Child Adolesc Psychiatry* 44(3): 240–248, doi:10.1097/00004583-200503000-00008.

NICE (2008) *Attention deficit hyperactivity disorder: Diagnosis and management. NICE Clinical Guidelines* [CG72], https://www.nice.org.uk/guidance/cg72.

Pliszka S (2015) Comorbid psychiatric disorders in children with ADHD. In Barkley R, ed. *Attention-deficit hyperactivity disorder*, 4th edn. New York, NY: Guilford Press, ISBN 978-1-4625-1772-5.

Silvestri R, Gagliano A, Calarese T et al. (2007) Ictal and interictal EEG abnormalities in ADHD children recorded over night by video-polysomnography. *Epilepsy Res* 75: 130–137, doi:10.1016/j.eplepsyres.2007.05.007.

Simonoff E, Taylor E, Baird G et al. (2013) Randomized controlled double-blind trial of optimal dose methylphenidate in children and adolescents with severe attention deficit hyperactivity disorder and intellectual disability. *J Child Psychol Psychiatry* 54(5): 527–535.

WHO (n.d.) *International Statistical Classification of Diseases and Related Health Problems*, 10th revision (ICD-10); available at www.who.int/classifications/icd/icdonlineversions/en/.

Chapter 5

Psychoeducation and behavioural management

David Daley

Case scenario

Frank and Michelle are young parents with three children. Their first son Tommy is 8 years of age. He has always been a helpful and easy-going child, does well at school and has lots of friends. Their second son, Jim, is 6 years of age and is completely different. Jims finds it very difficult to sit still for more than a few minutes. He is very distracted and has difficulty watching his favourite television programme for more than a few minutes. Jim is also very impulsive, and rarely thinks before he acts. This means that he constantly interrupts other people's conversations and has had several accidents, including pulling a saucepan of hot water onto himself when he was 3 years of age. Unlike his older brother who is very patient, Jim finds waiting very difficult. He always wants everything straight away, and would rather give up on a game or activity than wait his turn. Jim also has memory difficulties and finds it difficult to remember instructions or lists.

In many ways Jims behaves just like his younger brother Eddie, who is 2 and a half years' old, which frustrates his parents. Frank and Michelle consider themselves to be ordinary parents, neither strict nor lax, and take time and care in their parenting decisions. Jim's behaviour constantly makes them question their parenting skills and is a source of constant argument both between his parents and both sets of grandparents who all think he needs clear boundaries, stricter discipline and more punitive punishments such as 'a good clip around the ear'.

Frank and Michelle are not sure whether Jim's behaviour is the result of poor parenting skills, Jim's difficult temperament or simply lack of motivation. They often point to their other children as evidence of their parenting competence but are still struggling to convince themselves and others that they are not bad parents, although in public Jim often does make them look bad.

During their many late night discussions about Jim they often talk about the need to try and understand things from his point of view, to work out why paying attention or waiting his turn is so difficult, and react and respond differently to him than they do to their other children. Jims' teacher, at a recent parents' evening, confessed to having the same difficulties in school as Frank and Michelle experience at home.

What Frank and Michelle are slowly working out is that parenting a child with ADHD requires the parents to respond to that child in very specific ways, with little room for error. To put it another way, parents of children without ADHD can afford to be more lax, less consistent, and to make minor parenting errors without it impacting on their child's behaviour or development, but parents of children with ADHD rarely have any room for error.

This chapter aims to explore both psychoeducation (to enhance understanding of ADHD) and behavioural interventions that aim to develop proactive management strategies for ADHD in both the home and school context. Working with schools is discussed further in Chapter 10.

Introduction

Wymbs et al. (2015) explored parental treatment preferences in a sample of 445 parents accessing Canadian mental health services for their children with high levels of ADHD symptoms. The results showed that 58.7% of parents preferred individual behavioural management and were seeking to feel more informed about their child's problems and understand – as opposed to solve – their child's difficulties. A minority of parents (19.4%) preferred group behavioural management; these parents were mostly seeking strategies that would help them solve their child's problems. Nearly 22% of parents preferred a minimal information alternative such as psychoeducation; these parents reported the highest levels of depression and had children with the most complex problems. What the Wymbs et al. (2015) study demonstrates is that the parents of children with ADHD may be seeking different levels of services, and seeking help for different reasons. Therefore, a one size fits all approach is unlikely to be helpful or productive.

This chapter will introduce the reader to three different types of non-pharmacological intervention for ADHD: (1) psychoeducation, (2) behavioural parent training and

(3) school-based interventions. For each intervention approach we will consider three important questions:

- Why might this intervention approach work?

- What is currently available in the UK?

- Is there robust evidence to support the intervention?

The chapter will also discuss other important considerations such as parent-, child-, therapist- and service-specific factors that might limit the effectives of interventions, and offer some discussion of future directions in this area.

Psychoeducation

Why might psychoeducation be useful for ADHD?

Guidelines for ADHD support the use of psychoeducation programmes in the comprehensive management of ADHD (Ferrin & Taylor 2011). Psychoeducation has been defined as a systematic approach used to inform patients and their relatives about their illness, its underlying causes and treatment. The aim is to facilitate personal understanding, acceptance and coping. Psychoeducation interventions should be a sensitive, competent and sympathetic therapy, usually delivered in group settings, and should contain multiple sessions aimed at helping patients and carers to understand their complex difficulties.

Knowledge and understanding about ADHD are generally low in the general population, and children with ADHD, as well as their families, are at considerable risk of being confronted with stigma, prejudice and discrimination, as most people do not understand or appreciate why children with ADHD behave in the way that they do (Daley 2006). Without an adequate understanding of what drives the expression of ADHD symptoms, and why certain behaviours are functional rather than dysfunctional (Tarver et al. 2014), individuals with ADHD may perceive ADHD-related misbehaviours as reflecting personal flaws rather than their disorder (Fleischmann & Fleischmann 2012) while families will struggle to understand, support and advocate for their children with ADHD.

Montoya et al. (2011) were the first group to conduct a small systematic review of psychoeducation for ADHD focused on reviewing the results of seven studies that evaluated elements of psychoeducation. The results from the review were mixed, raised some questions about the evidence base for psychoeducation, but also highlighted the paucity of research in this area. Specifically, the results showed that psychoeducation was effective at reducing parental reports of ADHD symptoms in studies without a control group that assessed the ADHD symptoms before and after psychoeducation, but found no evidence that psychoeducation alone was effective when it was evaluated in a randomised controlled trial. There was some limited evidence that psychoeducation, when combined with other forms of non-pharmacological intervention, was effective (Ialongo et al. 1993). Looking beyond ADHD symptom control there was some evidence that psychoeducation alone helped to reduce reports of internalising symptoms, as well as parents' ability to manage their children's challenging behaviour.

Ferrin et al. (2014) report one of the most recent and largest randomised controlled trials comparing psychoeducation to counselling for children with ADHD. This study included 81 children aged 5–18 years with a diagnosis of ADHD (any subtype), recruited consecutively from a child psychiatric clinic in Spain. The psychoeducation programme consisted of twelve 90-minute group sessions and focused on helping parents to understand ADHD. The results demonstrated that in comparison to counselling, psychoeducation led to significant reductions in ADHD symptoms as measured by Conner's Parent Rated Scale, but had no significant effects on other child difficulties such as conduct problems. The effects persisted to 12 months follow-up for inattention, but not for hyperactive/impulsive symptoms. The lack of a maintenance effect for hyperactive/impulsive behaviours and any impact on other child difficulties does call into question the clinical utility of psychoeducation, as this study was as intensive as most behavioural interventions (which are reviewed in the following sections).

Behavioural interventions

Why might behavioural interventions be useful for ADHD?

Behavioural parenting interventions are recommended as first-line treatment options for the treatment of ADHD in childhood (NICE 2008) and have proven efficacy in reducing ADHD symptoms (Fabiano et al. 2009). As an alternative to drug therapy, behavioural intervention is considered a suitable first-level treatment for young children presenting with signs of ADHD (Daley 2006). Because of some evidence of the efficacy of these interventions with school-aged children with ADHD, an increasing number of empirical studies have, since the 1990s, evaluated the outcomes of parent training intervention for preschool-aged children with ADHD, and such interventions appear to be notably successful for this age group (Hartman et al. 2003). Following parent training intervention, improvements have been found in parent–child interaction (Pisterman et al. 1989), in compliance and on-task behaviour (Sonuga-Barke et al. 2001) and in parent-reported ADHD symptoms and child behaviour problems (Jones et al. 2007). However, concern has been raised as to whether such parenting interventions are sufficiently targeting ADHD symptoms, following meta-analysis evidence that effect sizes for behavioural interventions (including parenting interventions) drop to near zero when analysing data from informants who are probably blind to treatment allocation (Sonuga-Barke et al. 2013). These results question whether it is the effort of participating in an intervention rather than the content of the intervention that might make unblinded parents rate improvement in ADHD symptoms in their children at the end of intervention.

The strongest evidence for parent training comes from parents of preschool children (Box 5.1) and most probably reflects the premise that early intervention, before the child's transition to school and before the child's symptoms become associated with secondary problems such as academic failure, aggressive behaviour and conduct problems, provides the best opportunity to alter the developmental course of the disorder (Daley 2006).

When considering effective parent training treatments for ADHD during the preschool period, three interventions have been shown to be effective and are worthy of further discussion:

- *The New Forest Parent Training Programme* (NFPTP, Box 5.2; Sonuga-Barke et al. 2001)

- *The Triple P Positive Parenting Programme* (Triple-P, Box 5.3; Sanders et al. 2000)

- The Incredible Years Parent Training Programme (IYPTP, Box 5.4; Webster-Stratton & Hancock 1998; Jones et al. 2007, 2008)

Box 5.1: Preschool behavioural interventions

✓ The best evidence for behavioural interventions is in the preschool period.
✓ Why is this the optimal time?
  - neural plasticity
  - children spend the majority of their day with one or more of their parents
  - their symptoms are not yet associated with an antisocial tendency and school failure
✓ These factors can all combine to intervene to change the developmental trajectory of ADHD

Box 5.2: New Forest Parent Training Programme (NFPTP)

The NFPTP is a parent-based intervention package specifically designed to address the core symptoms of ADHD, as well as target key parenting skills.

The intervention entails eight 1-hour individual sessions delivered by specially trained therapists.

The programme focuses on four intervention components:

✓ Psycho-education
✓ Parent-child relationships, including positive parenting and extension of language to promote emotional self-regulation and play
✓ Behaviour training to encourage consistent limit setting
✓ Attention training to help parents work on improving their child's attention.

Source: Sonuga-Barke et al. (2001).

Box 5.3: The Triple P Positive Parenting Programme (Triple-P)

The standard version has an average of ten 1-hour sessions with a practitioner on an individual basis.

This programme teaches 17 core child management strategies including:

✓ Ten strategies to promote child competence and development (e.g. physical affection, attention and praise)

✓ Seven strategies to promote effective limit setting and manage disruptive behaviour (e.g. rule setting, directed discussion and time-out)

✓ A six-step planned activities routine is also introduced to parents to promote the generalisation and maintenance of parenting skills (e.g. planning ahead and joint decision-making)

Source: Sanders et al. (2000).

Box 5.4: The Incredible Years Parent Training Programme (IYPTP)

A group-based parenting intervention originally developed to treat conduct problems, available in a range of formats. Parents attend the group for 2.5 hours per week for 13–14 weeks. A 20- to 22-week ADHD-specific version is also available.

Skills taught on the 13–14 week basic programme include:

✓ How to establish a positive relationship with their child through play and child-centred activities

✓ Encouraging praise, reward and incentives for appropriate behaviours

✓ Guidance in the use of effective limit setting and clear instruction-giving

✓ Strategies for managing non-compliance

Parents acquire these skills through:

✓ Facilitator-led group discussion

✓ Brainstorming

✓ Videotape modelling

✓ Role-play

✓ Shared problem solving

✓ Rehearsal of taught intervention techniques through home assignments

Sources: Webster-Stratton & Hancock (1998) and Jones et al. (2007, 2008).

A 20- to 22-week ADHD specific version was used and evaluated by Webster-Stratton et al. (2011), which covered the same content as the 13- to 14-week version more slowly and included increased amounts of coaching for parents.

Why are these interventions successful at targeting ADHD?

While the NFPTP contains some of the key elements of a child and parents intervention, it has the added advantage of being directly informed by key aetiological theories of ADHD, and therefore addresses the core symptoms of ADHD (Sonuga-Barke et al. 2006). The programme contains psychoeducation about ADHD, games aimed at tackling cognitive dysregulation and inhibitory dysfunction, and strategies aimed at reducing delay aversion. However, despite the fact that Triple-P and IYPTP are interventions developed to treat and prevent conduct problems, they also appear to be effective at reducing ADHD symptoms in preschool children. This success may be attributed, at least in part, to the sound theoretical grounding of these interventions. Effective parent training interventions draw from the principles of social learning theory and highlight the reciprocal nature of the parent–child interaction. Parents acquire behaviour management techniques, such as effective use of praise, using language to describe feelings, giving clear, concise instructions, effective limit setting and the use of non-violent discipline techniques, all within the context of positive, sensitive and responsive parenting (Box 5.5). It is well documented that sensitive, responsive parenting in the early years provides the foundation for the development of child self-regulation skills (Hughes et al. 2009). Children with ADHD have particular difficulties with self-regulation skills such as listening, attending and controlling their temper (Daley & Thompson 2007). Therefore, providing parents with effective strategies, tailored to their child's individual needs, promotes child self-regulation and can be instrumental in reducing the symptoms of ADHD. The inclusion of strategies to promote more effective coping, problem solving and communication skills may also help parents to deal with the day-to-day stressors associated with parenting a child with ADHD.

Box 5.5: Helpful techniques that can be acquired in parent ADHD management courses

Helpful techniques:

✓ Effective use of praise
✓ Using language to describe feelings
✓ Giving clear, concise instructions
✓ Effective limit setting
✓ Use of non-violent discipline techniques
✓ Effective coping strategies
✓ Problem solving
✓ Communication skills

All within the context of positive, sensitive and responsive parenting.

Is there a robust evidence base to support parent training for ADHD?

The evidence base supporting the interventions reviewed above has several methodological issues that warrant further discussion. First, in terms of the measures used to assess the symptoms of preschool ADHD, the NFPTP trial was particularly robust. The evaluation measured child ADHD symptoms using the Parental Account of Children's Symptoms (Taylor et al. 1991) – a well-validated structured clinical interview – as well as an objective observation measure of child attention and task switching (Sonuga-Barke et al. 2001). The evaluation of the IYPTP programme for ADHD has been less robust. It is worth noting that the first IYPTP evaluation for ADHD was conducted within the context of a larger trial – the North Wales Sure Start Trial. The trial evaluated the IYPTP on a community sample of preschool children at risk of developing conduct problems (Hutchings et al. 2007) and the evaluation of children with conduct problems and ADHD relied solely on parental report. A second study (Webster-Stratton et al. 2011) was a much better prospective study, and although it did include blinded objective measures of ADHD, they did not show any change in response to treatment. To date, the one study that has evaluated Triple-P is relatively weak, because it relied heavily on self-report and the ADHD outcome is a factor score created from a conduct problem scale (Daley et al. 2009).

Second, the NFPTP evidence base is particularly strong as it was compared against a comparison counselling intervention group (Sonuga-Barke et al. 2001), in addition to a standard waiting list control group, as well as treatment as usual (Thompson et al. 2009). With such a design, one can be more confident in concluding that the intervention outcomes are due to the components of the intervention as opposed to contact with therapists/services, as well as double check that the intervention is better than what is routinely used in clinics. Although the Triple-P evaluation did examine two intervention groups against a waiting list control group, one of these interventions was simply a more enhanced version of the other, and therefore both shared much of their therapeutic content. The IYPTP trials only compared the intervention group with a standard control group.

Third, NFPTP and Triple-P are relatively brief interventions (eight 1-hour sessions for NFPTP and 8 hours of group intervention and 90 minutes of telephone support for Triple-P). However, for IYPTP the intensity of intervention was much greater, with 12 group sessions (24–30 hours) for Jones et al. (2007) and at least 20 group sessions (40 hours) for the parent and 20 group sessions (40 hours) for the child in Webster-Stratton et al. (2011). The need for such an intensive intervention may make IYPTP unfeasible within routine clinical care in the UK.

Finally, establishing the long-term stability of intervention outcomes is of particular importance. There is some evidence to suggest that parent training programmes are not entirely successful with every family, especially in the long term. Unfortunately, the positive effects of many intervention programmes decline rapidly after the intervention. In this context, the IYPTP evaluation was particularly robust, demonstrating 12- (Webster-Stratton et al. 2013) and 18-month stability of intervention effects (Jones et al. 2008), whereas the Triple-P reported 12-month stability (Bor et al. 2002), and for NFPTP, outcome stability was only reported 15 weeks after programme completion (Sonuga-Barke et al. 2001).

The evidence base for parent training with older children with ADHD is much weaker, with fewer clear results, as there is a degree of variability in its effectiveness in the management of childhood ADHD (Anastopoulos et al. 1993). Age again appears to be a factor, with interventions being more effective for younger children with problems relating to compliance, rule-following, defiance and aggression. Sonuga-Barke et al. (2013) explored the efficacy of non-pharmacological intervention for children with ADHD, looking at ADHD outcomes only. A consistent pattern emerged, with small to moderate effect size improvements reported by individuals most proximal to the receipt of treatment (MPROX; usually parents) and much smaller and usually non-significant effects sizes from more probably blinded informants (PBLIND) across psychological and dietary interventions. This led Sonuga-Barke et al. (2013) to conclude that more evidence was needed before non-pharmacological interventions could be considered evidence-based interventions for ADHD symptom change. A follow-up series of meta-analyses based on updated versions of the Sonuga-Barke meta-analysis explored different non-pharmacological interventions in greater detail, and looked beyond just ADHD symptoms (Daley et al. 2014.) Sonuga-Barke's distinction between MPROX and PBLIND with respect to ADHD symptom change was replicated, but significant MPROX and PBLIND improvements in conduct problems, positive and negative parenting, and MPROX improvements in child social skills, academic attainment, as well as parental self-concept were demonstrated (Daley et al. 2014). A large proportion of the samples in most papers included in the analysis reported considerable parental mental health difficulties, and the analysis did not demonstrate improvement in this. Meta-regression also showed larger effect sizes in studies with younger children, suggesting that the age of the child may influence the likelihood of success.

Thus, psychosocial intervention is a valuable treatment option, especially during pre-school years. Meta-analysis may suggest that behavioural interventions have little success in changing core ADHD symptoms, but there is clear evidence that they do improve a number of other important outcomes (Box 5.6). What is urgently needed is robust evidence that parent training is effective in routine clinical samples of children aged between 6 and 12 years with a diagnosis of ADHD.

Chapter 12 describes a parent management group used in one team with extremely positive feedback from families who attended.

Box 5.6: Psychosocial intervention in ADHD

✓ Psychosocial intervention is a valuable treatment option, especially during the preschool years
✓ The lack of an effect recorded by blinded observers in the Daley et al. (2014) meta-analysis may suggest that behavioural interventions do not change core ADHD symptoms
✓ There is clear evidence that psychosocial interventions improve parenting and reduce conduct problems

Psychoeducation and behavioural management in school

Practical advice around school-based intervention is presented in Chapter 10. Here we will consider some of the research evidence.

Why might psychoeducation and behavioural management work in schools?

The impact of ADHD on school life is seen through two different routes. Research evidence clearly demonstrates the impact of ADHD symptoms on academic attainment (Birchwood & Daley 2010; Sayal et al. 2015) as well as the fact that children with ADHD often become a focus for classroom disruption (Tarver et al. 2014).

Montoya et al. (2011), in their systematic review (discussed previously in the 'Behavioural interventions' section), also considered the impact of psychoeducation alone on academic achievement. Three studies explored the impact of either parent- or teacher-focused psychoeducation on academic outcomes (Ialongo et al. 1993; Miranda et al. 2002; Svanborg et al. 2009). The results demonstrated that only teacher-focused psychoeducation (Miranda et al. 2002) improved academic outcomes, which makes intuitive sense.

Hodgson and colleagues (2012) conducted a meta-analysis of non-pharmacological interventions for ADHD and concluded that there was no evidence to support interventions in school settings. However, this conclusion was based on averaging effect sizes across a range of outcomes and included effect sizes that were sometimes based on only one study. In contrast, Moore et al. (2015) and Richardson et al. (2015) both report results from a study that conducted an overarching synthesis of four systematic reviews including 138 studies focused on non-pharmacological interventions for ADHD in school settings. The results from Moore et al. (2015) and Richardson et al. (2015) highlighted evidence for the impact of school-focused intervention on reducing inattention and hyperactive/impulsive symptoms when measured using neurocognitive tests, as well as evidence of improvements on teachers' reports of inattention but not hyperactive/impulsive symptoms. There was also some evidence for the impact of school-focused interventions on improving externalising behaviour. In terms of academic attainment there was evidence of a beneficial effect of intervention on teacher perceptions of scholastic adjustment and some evidence of improvements in standardised achievement. Improvement in standardised achievement, however, has been suggested to be the most important outcome for both teachers and pupils (Langberg et al. 2011).

Some other key considerations

Moderators of outcome: For whom do behavioural interventions work best?

Van Der Oord and Daley (2014) explored the moderators of outcome for behavioural interventions for ADHD. There are only two studies assessing moderation for behavioural intervention within ADHD samples. The intensity and scope of both these interventions differ: the Multi Modal Study of ADHD (MTA) behavioural intervention was multimodal and intense, while the other intervention resembles the behavioural parent interventions often used in clinical practice, i.e. outpatient, short-term and unimodal.

For outpatient, short-term, behavioural parent interventions, comorbidity and parenting self-efficacy (of both mother and father) and paternal ADHD symptoms are important indicators of treatment success. Parents with high self-efficacy, fathers with high levels of ADHD symptoms and children with only one or no comorbid conditions are most likely to benefit from these parent interventions. Parents that are confident of providing parenting techniques may benefit most from behavioural parent training. Also, with regard to the possibility of breaking the coercive cycle, for those with the least comorbid problem behaviour, it may be easier to break the coercive cycle. Somewhat counterintuitively, children with fathers with high levels of ADHD symptoms respond best to additive behavioural treatment, which may be related to the fact that there is more room for improvement for the behavioural techniques taught in the interventions for these fathers.

Richardson et al. (2015) explored the role of moderators of outcome for school-based interventions using meta-regression. Their results showed that intervention-related improvements in inattention, hyperactive/impulsive behaviour or externalising symptoms were influenced by participant characteristics, components of intervention (study skills, contingency training, self-regulation) and intervention delivery (context, provider, time setting or duration). The absence of any moderators of outcome suggests that the success of these interventions can be achieved without any particular concern about the type, mode or context of school-based intervention.

Mediators of outcome: what indirect effects help us to understand how behavioural interventions impact outcomes?

Very little is known about mediation in the context of interventions for ADHD. The reduction of ineffective and negative parenting appears to be an important mediator of behavioural intervention outcome and thus may need to be targeted and monitored specifically during intervention, especially for parents with ADHD themselves (Sonuga-Barke et al. 2002). For the improvement of academic skills of children with ADHD through behavioural intervention, enhancing organisation skills during intervention is important, especially in order to achieve better academic functioning at school.

Implementation fidelity

Very little is known about the impact of implementation fidelity (how well the therapist delivers the intervention) on psychoeducation and behavioural interventions for ADHD. For conduct disorder, Eames et al. (2009) demonstrated that implementation fidelity predicted the outcome for preschool children at risk of conduct disorder whose parents were engaging in behavioural parent training. In a follow-up study (Eames et al. 2010), a more detailed exploration of the relationship between implementation fidelity and outcome demonstrated that the skills that were modelled most by therapists in the group parent training sessions were the skills that parents demonstrated in interactions with their children during a structured interaction play task at 6-month follow-up visits. However, it is clear that the evidence for the impact of implementation fidelity on outcome underlines the need for intervention-specific training and supervision for the individuals responsible for delivering interventions.

Mode of delivery and service considerations

Group versus individual intervention

The current recommendations from the National Institute of Health and Clinical Excellence for ADHD (NICE 2008) direct therapists towards group parent training interventions based on the principles of social learning theory. Although there is evidence to suggest that interventions based on social learning theory are effective for children with or at risk of ADHD (Webster-Stratton et al. 2011; Jones et al. 2007, 2008), there is no evidence to suggest that group intervention is better than individual intervention. Parents of children with ADHD often display symptoms of ADHD themselves and often struggle more with the organisational challenges of attending group-based interventions. A recent study by Sonuga-Barke et al. (submitted) explored the relative efficacy of an individual home-based parenting programme for ADHD (the NFPTP) against a group-based intervention (IYPTP) and compared them both to treatment as usual for a large group of hard-to-engage and difficult-to-treat parents of preschool children at risk of ADHD. The results suggested no clear advantage of the home-based intervention over the group-based intervention in terms of symptoms outcome, but clear evidence that the individual intervention was more cost-effective, and some evidence as indexed by engagement rates of parents that individual home-based intervention was preferred by parents.

Social skills training

There is little evidence to support the use of currently available social skills training for children with ADHD alone, but there may be a place for this when there is comorbid autism spectrum disorder or social communication disorder.

Cognitive-behavioural therapy (CBT)

A number of therapies based on CBT have been developed for use with children and young people. Evidence of success in treating ADHD symptoms is not robust, but CBT may be indicated to manage comorbid problems.

Anger management

Parents frequently ask about 'anger management'. In children there is little evidence of success with anger management techniques. If the child/young person is requesting help, there may be more hope of improvement.

Box 5.7 summarises the recommendations in the NICE Guideline around behavioural management.

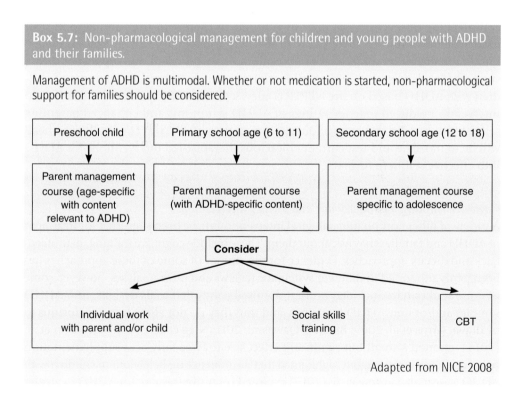

Box 5.7: Non-pharmacological management for children and young people with ADHD and their families.

Management of ADHD is multimodal. Whether or not medication is started, non-pharmacological support for families should be considered.

| Preschool child | Primary school age (6 to 11) | Secondary school age (12 to 18) |

| Parent management course (age-specific with content relevant to ADHD) | Parent management course (with ADHD-specific content) | Parent management course specific to adolescence |

Consider

| Individual work with parent and/or child | Social skills training | CBT |

Adapted from NICE 2008

Generic versus specialised behavioural intervention

A recent study by Abikoff et al. (2015) explored the relative efficacy of a generic social learning theory-based intervention for ADHD (Helping the Noncompliant Child; Cunningham et al. 2004) against a specialised ADHD intervention, the NFPTP (Thompson et al. 2009). Both interventions were delivered as individual home-based programmes to American parents of children at risk of ADHD and compared to a treatment-as-usual group. The results clearly demonstrated that both interventions were significantly better than treatment as usual, but specialised parent training for ADHD in this study was not significantly better than a more generic parenting intervention.

Self-help interventions

Despite the availability of effective interventions, the prevalence of ADHD creates a need that far exceeds available personnel and resources. In many parts of the UK, parents often have to travel long distances to access services provided at inconvenient times, leading to high levels of non-engagement or non-completion. A Cochrane review (Montgomery et al. 2006) concluded that self-help interventions were worth considering in clinical practice targeting child behaviour problems. They could reduce the amount of time therapists have to devote to each case, increase access to intervention, and release clinician time to concentrate on more complex cases. For families, self-administered interventions significantly reduce or eliminate costs, transport and timing difficulties. Families can complete the intervention in their own home, in their own time and at their own pace. Evidence supports the efficacy of self-help intervention for childhood behaviour problems, either on its own or in combination with telephone support or media support (Sanders et al. 2007). A pilot trial of a self-help book for parents of children with ADHD based on the NFPTP (Daley & O'Brien 2013) showed that self-help intervention reduced parents' ratings of ADHD symptoms and enhanced parenting self-esteem, but did not change objective measures of ADHD. The challenge ahead will be to translate and test current efficacious therapist-led interventions for ADHD into effective self-help formats.

Cognitive training, neurofeedback and dietary interventions

A variety of other non-pharmacological interventions have been suggested for treatment of ADHD and families may ask about them. These include cognitive training, neurofeedback and dietary approaches. Evidence for the efficacy of some of these approaches has been partly supported in different systematic reviews and meta-analyses; however, some of these studies have included non-randomised controlled trials designs, non-ADHD samples and/or non-ADHD outcomes, and thus they do not allow firm conclusions to be drawn (Arns et al. 2009; Bloch & Qawasmi, 2011; Nigg et al. 2012). Stevenson et al. (2014) reported a small but significant effect size for free fatty acid supplementation based on PBLIND ratings, but highlighted that its influence on behaviour in children with ADHD was small. Cortese et al. (2015) explored cognitive training for ADHD in greater detail and found that despite improving working memory performance, cognitive training had limited effects on ADHD symptoms according to assessments based on PBLIND measures. Similarly, evidence from well-controlled trials with PBLIND outcomes failed to support neurofeedback as an effective treatment for ADHD (Cortese et al. 2016).

Future directions

There follows a brief description of a few current projects that will no doubt impact future interventions for ADHD. I am currently involved in a research consortium that is developing an online version of the NFPTP, to provide an entirely digital version of this evidence-based face-to-face intervention. Although trial evidence for its effectiveness is years away, in all likelihood it will only be successful for highly motivated parents with few other problems and for children with lower levels of ADHD-related impairment. However, the hope is that greater use of online intervention for some will allow greater access and more resources in the clinic for parents who may not be suitable for online intervention. Online delivery of social-learning-theory-based interventions for conduct problems are already available and evidence based (Sanders et al. 2012).

The delivery of standard psychoeducation advice for ADHD is beginning to be incorporated into a downloadable app (Kumaragama & Dasanayake 2015) and over the next few years I would anticipate an explosion in their availability. The challenge for clinicians will be to ensure that their patients engage with the 'good' ones and avoid the 'bad' ones.

Summary

- Psychoeducation about ADHD may be helpful for parents, but services need to be mindful that psychoeducation alone is often as intensive and costly as other forms of non-pharmacological intervention.

- Behavioural interventions for ADHD are effective at reducing parental ratings and more objective reports of conduct problems, parenting practices as well as parental ratings of ADHD symptoms.

- Developmental age may be important, with better results achieved for studies targeting younger children.

- There is some evidence for the impact of interventions for ADHD on educational outcomes and school attainment, but the evidence is limited.

- Very little is known about moderators of mediations of intervention for ADHD.

- Mode of delivery is also important to consider, with recent trial evidence suggesting that both group and individual interventions achieve comparable results, but individual intervention is less costly.

References

Abikoff HB, Thompson M, Laver-Bradbury C et al. (2015) Parent training for preschool ADHD: A randomized controlled trial of specialized and generic programs. *J Child Psychol Psychiatry* 56(6): 618–631.

Anastopoulos AD, Shelton TL, DuPaul GJ et al. (1993) Parent training for attention-deficit hyperactivity disorder: Its impact on parent functioning. *J Abnorm Child Psychol* 21(5): 581–596.

Arns M, de Ridder S, Strehl U, Breteler M, Coenen A (2009) Efficacy of neurofeedback treatment in ADHD: The effects on inattention, impulsivity and hyperactivity: a meta-analysis. *Clin EEG Neurosci* 40(3): 180–189.

Birchwood J, Daley D (2012) Brief report: The impact of attention deficit hyperactivity disorder (ADHD) symptoms on academic performance in an adolescent community sample. *J Adolesc* 35(1): 225–231.

Bloch MH, Qawasmi A (2011) Omega-3 fatty acid supplementation for the treatment of children with attention-deficit/hyperactivity disorder symptomatology: Systematic review and meta-analysis. *J Am Acad Child Adolesc Psychiatry* 50(10): 991–1000.

Bor W, Sanders M, Markie-Dadds C (2002) The effects of the Triple P-Positive Parenting Program on preschool children with co-occurring disruptive behavior and attentional/hyperactive difficulties. *J Abnorm Child Psychol* 30(6): 571–587.

Cortese S, Ferrin M, Brandeis D et al. (2015) Cognitive training for attention-deficit/hyperactivity disorder: meta-analysis of clinical and neuropsychological outcomes from randomized controlled trials. *J Am Acad Child Adolesc Psychiatry* 54(3): 164–174.

Cortese S, Ferrin M, Brandeis D et al. (2016) Neurofeedback for attention-deficit/hyperactivity disorder: Meta-analysis of clinical and neuropsychological outcomes from randomized controlled trials. *J Am Acad Child Adolesc Psychiatry* 55(6): 444–455.

Cunningham CE, McHolm A, Boyle MH, Patel S (2004) Behavioral and emotional adjustment, family functioning, academic performance, and social relationships in children with selective mutism. *J Child Psychol Psychiatry* 45(8): 1363–1372.

Daley D (2006) Attention deficit hyperactivity disorder: A review of the essential facts. *Child: Care Health Dev* 32(2): 193–204.

Daley D, Thompson M (2007) Parent training for ADHD in preschool children. *Adv ADHD* 2(1): 11–16.

Daley D, Jones K, Hutchings J, Thompson M (2009) Attention deficit hyperactivity disorder in pre-school children: Current findings, recommended interventions and future directions. *Child: Care Health Dev* 35(6): 754–766.

Daley D, O'Brien M (2013) A small-scale randomized controlled trial of the self-help version of the New Forest Parent Training Programme for children with ADHD symptoms. *Eur Child Adolesc Psychiatry* 22(9): 543–552.

Daley D, Van der Oord S, Ferrin M et al. (2014) Behavioral interventions in attention-deficit/ hyperactivity disorder: A meta-analysis of randomized controlled trials across multiple outcome domains. *J Am Acad Child Adolesc Psychiatry* 53(8): 835–847.

Eames C, Daley D, Hutchings J et al. (2009) Treatment fidelity as a predictor of behaviour change in parents attending group-based parent training. *Child: Care Health Dev* 35(5): 603–612.

Eames C, Daley D, Hutchings J et al. (2010) The impact of group leaders' behaviour on parents acquisition of key parenting skills during parent training. *Behav Res Ther* 48(12): 1221–1226.

Fabiano GA, Pelham WE, Coles EK, Gnagy EM, Chronis-Tuscano A, O'Connor BC (2009) A meta-analysis of behavioral treatments for attention-deficit/hyperactivity disorder. *Clin Psychol Rev* 29(2): 129–140.

Ferrin M, Moreno-Granados JM, Salcedo-Marin MD, Ruiz-Veguilla M, Perez-Ayala V, Taylor E (2014) Evaluation of a psychoeducation programme for parents of children and adolescents with ADHD: Immediate and long-term effects using a blind randomized controlled trial. *Eur Child Adolesc Psychiatry* 23(8): 637–647.

Ferrin M, Taylor E (2011) Child and caregiver issues in treatment of attention deficit-hyperactivity disorder: Education, adherence and treatment choice. *Fut Neurol* 6: 399–413.

Fleischmann A, Fleischmann RH (2012) Advantages of an ADHD diagnosis in adulthood evidence from online narratives. *Qualitat Health Res* 22(11): 1486–1496.

Hartman RR, Stage SA, Webster-Stratton C (2003) A growth curve analysis of parent training outcomes: Examining the influence of child risk factors (inattention, impulsivity, and hyperactivity problems), parental and family risk factors. *J Child Psychol Psychiatry* 44(3): 388–398.

Hodgson K, Hutchinson AD, Denson L (2012) Nonpharmacological treatments for ADHD: A meta-analytic review. *J Atten Disord* 18(4): 275–282.

Hughes CH, Ensor RA (2009) How do families help or hinder the emergence of early executive function? *New Direct Child Adolesc Dev* 2009(123): 35–50.

Hutchings J, Bywater T, Daley D et al. (2007) Parenting intervention in Sure Start services for children at risk of developing conduct disorder: pragmatic randomised controlled trial. *BMJ* 334(7595): 678.

Ialongo NS, Horn WF, Pascoe JM et al. (1993) The effects of a multimodal intervention with attention-deficit hyperactivity disorder children: A 9-month follow-up. *J Am Acad Child Adolesc Psychiatry* 32(1): 182–189.

Jones K, Daley D, Hutchings J, Bywater T, Eames C (2007) Efficacy of the Incredible Years Basic Parent Training Programme as an early intervention for children with conduct problems and ADHD. *Child: Care Health Dev* 33(6): 749–756.

Jones K, Daley D, Hutchings J, Bywater T, Eames C (2008) Efficacy of the Incredible Years Programme as an early intervention for children with conduct problems and ADHD: Long-term follow-up. *Child: Care Health Dev* 34(3): 380–390.

Kumaragama K, Dasanayake P (2015) iOS Applications (apps) for attention deficit hyperactivity disorder (ADHD/ADD): A preliminary investigation from Australia. *J Mob Technol Med* 4(2): 33–39.

Langberg JM, Vaughn AJ, Williamson P, Epstein JN, Girio-Herrera E, Becker SP (2011) Refinement of an organizational skills intervention for adolescents with ADHD for implementation by school mental health providers. *School Mental Health* 3(3): 143–155.

Miranda A, Presentación MJ, Soriano M (2002) Effectiveness of a school-based multicomponent program for the treatment of children with ADHD. *J Learning Disabil* 35(6): 547–563.

Montgomery P, Bjornstad G, Dennis J (2006) Media-based behavioural treatments for behavioural problems in children. *Cochrane Database Syst Rev* 1.

Montoya A, Colom F, Ferrin M (2011) Is psychoeducation for parents and teachers of children and adolescents with ADHD efficacious? A systematic literature review. *Eur Psychiatry* 26(3): 166–175.

Moore DA, Richardson M, Gwernan-Jones R et al. (2015) Non-pharmacological interventions for ADHD in school settings: An overarching synthesis of systematic reviews. *J Atten Disord* 2015 Mar 9. pii: 1087054715573994.

National Collaborating Centre for Mental Health (UK). Attention-Deficit/Hyperactivity Disorder: Diagnosis and Management of ADHD in Children, Young People and Adults. British Psychological Society (UK); 2009.

NICE (2008) *Attention deficit hyperactivity disorder: Diagnosis and management. NICE Clinical Guidelines* [CG72], https://www.nice.org.uk/guidance/cg72.

Nigg JT, Lewis K, Edinger T, Falk M (2012) Meta-analysis of attention-deficit/hyperactivity disorder or attention-deficit/hyperactivity disorder symptoms, restriction diet, and synthetic food color additives. *J Am Acad Child Adolesc Psychiatry* 51(1): 86–97.

Pisterman S, McGrath P, Firestone P, Goodman JT, Webster I, Mallory R (1989) Outcome of parent-mediated treatment of preschoolers with attention deficit disorder with hyperactivity. *J Consult Clin Psychol* 57(5): 628.

Richardson M, Moore DA, Gwernan-Jones R et al. (2015) *Non-pharmacological interventions for attention-deficit/hyperactivity disorder (ADHD) delivered in school settings: Systematic reviews of quantitative and qualitative research.* Winchester: Health Technology Assessment.

Sanders MR, Markie-Dadds C, Tully LA, Bor W (2000) The Triple P-positive parenting program: A comparison of enhanced, standard, and self-directed behavioral family intervention for parents of children with early onset conduct problems. *J Consult Clin Psychol* 68(4): 624.

Sanders MR, Bor W, Morawska A (2007) Maintenance of treatment gains: A comparison of enhanced, standard, and self-directed Triple P-Positive Parenting Program. *J Abnorm Child Psychol* 35(6): 983–998.

Sanders MR, Baker S, Turner KM (2012) A randomized controlled trial evaluating the efficacy of Triple P Online with parents of children with early-onset conduct problems. *Behav Res Ther* 50(11): 675–684.

Sayal K, Washbrook E, Propper C (2015) Childhood behaviour problems and academic outcomes in adolescence: Longitudinal population-based study. *J Am Acad Child Adolesc Psychiatry* 54(5): 360–368.

Sonuga-Barke EJ, Daley D, Thompson M, Laver-Bradbury C, Weeks A (2001) Parent-based therapies for preschool attention-deficit/hyperactivity disorder: A randomized, controlled trial with a community sample. *J Am Acad Child Adolesc Psychiatry* 40(4): 402–408.

Sonuga-Barke E, Daley D, Thompson M (2002) Does maternal ADHD reduce the effectiveness of parent training for preschool children's ADHD? *J Am Acad Child Adolesc Psychiatry* 41(6): 696–702.

Sonuga-Barke EJ, Thompson M, Abikoff H, Klein R, Brotman LM (2006) Nonpharmacological interventions for preschoolers with ADHD: The case for specialized parent training. *Infants Young Children* 19(2): 142–153.

Sonuga-Barke EJS, Brandeis D, Cortese S et al. (2013) Nonpharmacological interventions for ADHD: Systematic review and meta-analyses of randomized controlled trials of dietary and psychological treatments. *Am J Psychiatr* 170(3): 275–289.

Stevenson J, Buitelaar J, Cortese S et al. (2014) Research review: The role of diet in the treatment of attention-deficit/hyperactivity disorder–an appraisal of the evidence on efficacy and recommendations on the design of future studies. *J Child Psychol Psychiatry* 55(5): 416–427.

Svanborg P, Thernlund G, Gustafsson PA, Hägglöf B, Poole L, Kadesjö B (2009) Efficacy and safety of atomoxetine as add-on to psychoeducation in the treatment of attention deficit/hyperactivity disorder. *Eur Child Adolesc Psychiatry* 18(4): 240–249.

Tarver J, Daley D, Sayal K (2014) Attention-deficit hyperactivity disorder (ADHD): An updated review of the essential facts. *Child: Care Health Dev* 40(6): 762–774.

Taylor E, Sandberg S, Thorley G, Giles S (1991) *The epidemiology of childhood hyperactivity*. Oxford: Oxford University Press.

Thompson MJ, Laver-Bradbury C, Ayres M et al. (2009) A small-scale randomized controlled trial of the revised new forest parenting programme for preschoolers with attention deficit hyperactivity disorder. *Eur Child Adolesc Psychiatry* 18(10): 605–616.

Van der Oord S, Daley D (2014). Moderation and mediation of treatment outcomes for children with ADHD. In: Maric M, Prins P, Ollendick T (eds) *Moderators and mediators of youth treatment outcomes*. New York, NY: Oxford University Press.

Webster-Stratton C, Hancock L (1998) Parent training for young children with conduct problems. Content, methods and therapeutic process. In: Schaefer CE (eds) *Handbook of parent training*. New York, NY: Wiley, pp. 98–152.

Webster-Stratton CH, Reid MJ, Beauchaine T (2011) Combining parent and child training for young children with ADHD. *J Clin Child Adolesc Psychol* 40(2): 191–203.

Webster-Stratton C, Reid MJ, Beauchaine TP (2013) One-year follow-up of combined parent and child intervention for young children with ADHD. *J Clin Child Adolesc Psychol* 42(2): 251–261.

Wymbs FA, Cunningham CE, Chen Y et al. (2015) Examining parents' preferences for group and individual parent training for children with ADHD symptoms. *J Clin Child Adolesc Psychol* 43: 614–631.

Chapter 6

Medication: the drugs available to treat ADHD

Peter Hill

This chapter considers the currently available medications for the treatment of ADHD. It will describe the different medications and what is known about their modes of action, efficacy and side effects. Chapter 7 will discuss their use in clinical practice.

Medication for ADHD has a long history, effectively dating back to Charles Bradley's observation in 1937 of the beneficial effect of racemic amfetamine on noisy, badly behaved children. This was an incidental finding, and the use of stimulant medication for hyperactive children did not become widely established until the 1960s, predominantly in the USA. Although dexamfetamine had been used for years to treat hyperactivity in a small number of children, the main increase in the use of medication for hyperactivity disorders followed the Food and Drug Administration approval of methylphenidate for use in childhood in the USA in 1962 and the evolution of the attention deficit disorder (ADD)/ADHD concept from 1980 onwards. In the UK, methylphenidate, hitherto available on a named patient basis, was placed on general release in 1991, and a sharp increase in prescription rate followed, although this had plateaued by 2006 (Holden et al. 2013).

Given the universal acceptance of the role of the catecholamine neurotransmitters, dopamine, and noradrenaline in the pathophysiology of ADHD, it is not surprising that all medications exert their effect by enhancing and prolonging the action of noradrenaline and dopamine at the central nervous system (CNS) neuronal synapse (Box 6.1), particularly in the basal ganglia and prefrontal cortex. There are minor differences between

Box 6.1: Interneuronal synapse in the CNS, illustrating the site of action of ADHD medications

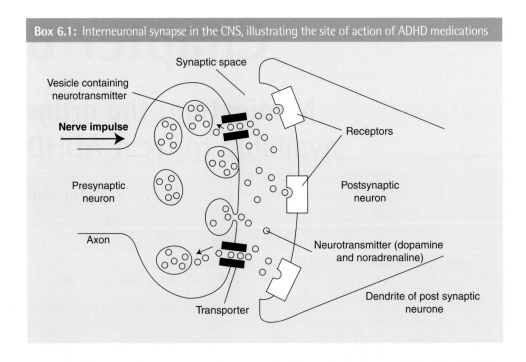

Box 6.2: ADHD medications and their modes of action

Stimulants

- Methylphenidate $\longrightarrow$ Increases DA and NA in synapse by blocking the DA and NA transporter and may increase output

- Amfetamine $\longrightarrow$ Increases DA and NA by blocking the DA and NA transporters and increasing output

Selective NA reuptake inhibitor

- Atomoxetine $\longrightarrow$ Increases NA and DA by blocking the NA transporter

α_2-Agonist

- Clonidine $\longrightarrow$ Engages $\alpha_{2a,}$ α_{2b}-and α_{2c} adrenergic receptors equally

Selective α_{2a}-agonist

- Guanfacine $\longrightarrow$ Selective for the α_{2a}-adrenergic receptor

While the indirect actions of stimulants and atomoxetine increase catecholamine availability in the synapse, the α_2-agonists work directly on receptors

Notes: DA, dopamine; NA, noradrenaline.

them in how this is achieved, and the mechanisms for doing so are less straightforward than sometimes assumed.

Conventionally, medications for ADHD are simply divided into stimulants and non-stimulants, but this is becoming an unhelpful simplification and it will be more helpful to subdivide non-stimulants further, ideally according to pharmacological action (Box 6.2).

Stimulant medications

The stimulants methylphenidate and dexamfetamine are by far the most efficacious and widely used agents. Both are controlled drugs: in the UK they are listed under Class B (Misuse of Drugs Act 1971), Schedule 2 (Misuse of Drugs Regulations 2001). In the USA they are Schedule II controlled substances. When used for the treatment of ADHD in childhood, the risk of addiction or misuse is minimal, particularly when sustained release preparations are used.

Methylphenidate is specifically recommended by all practice guidelines as the usual starting medication for ADHD unless contraindicated. In the USA either methylphenidate or dexamfetamine are recommended as initial options.

Both stimulants have similar side effects and are broadly equivalent in potency as far as group studies are concerned. Nevertheless, in individual head-to-head studies, dexamfetamine often has a slight advantage for potency (Hodgkins et al. 2012). The reason for this mild discrepancy probably lies in the important differences when individuals are considered, as there are children who will respond only or preferentially to each one and in some work preferential response to dexamfetamine is slightly more common. In a comparative review of studies (Arnold 2000), 61% of stimulant responders respond equally well to either stimulant, about 23% respond better to dexamfetamine and 16% to methylphenidate (I have recalculated the original percentages after omitting the small number who responded to neither).

The importance of this is exemplified by the work of Ramtvedt et al. (2013) who trialled all referrals to an ADHD service on both methylphenidate and dexamfetamine. Echoing Arnold's figures, although 53% of their children responded equally well to both stimulants, 39% responded favourably only to one. In this study, preference rates were equal between methylphenidate and dexamfetamine. Overall, simply trialling a single stimulant produced a favourable response in 72% of patients. When both stimulants were tried and the better one selected, the overall positive treatment response rate climbed to 92%. These findings on individual differences on preferentiality have enormous importance for clinical practice.

In order to explain such differences in individual responses it helps to examine the differences in pharmacological action between the two stimulants. Nevertheless, the common ground is important. Both have similar molecular shapes that resemble the two principal CNS catecholamine neurotransmitters – dopamine and noradrenaline – thus enabling competition for monoamine receptor sites and intracellular storage. Both stimulants can activate trace amine associated receptor 1 (TAAR1), which in turn modulates membrane monoamine transporters.

Methylphenidate
The usual form of methylphenidate is a racemic mixture (50:50 d,l-threo-methylphenidate), although the l-isomer has little, if any, effect. An isolated preparation of the d-isomer (dexmethylphenidate) is available in the USA and a few other countries, but not in Europe, apart from Switzerland.

The most prominent action of methylphenidate is blockade of the activity of the dopamine transporter (DAT) molecule on the presynaptic neuron membrane at the synapse. This transporter enables reuptake from the synaptic cleft of previously released dopamine. The dopamine transporter is not very selective and will also reuptake noradrenaline. Methylphenidate acts to block reuptake simply by occupying the transporter.

It is generally asserted that this DAT blockade is the way in which methylphenidate works, enhancing dopamine activity by increasing its quantity and duration in the synaptic cleft so that it is more available to post-synaptic receptors. Yet Heal (e.g. Heal et al. 2011) has challenged this, because a synthesised (but not marketed) pure dopamine reuptake blocker is ineffective in ADHD. Additionally, in rat studies, the sheer size and prompt efflux of dopamine and noradrenaline caused by methylphenidate exceeds and does not look like a classic reuptake inhibitor action. Although it is true that methylphenidate does indeed block reuptake of dopamine by the presynaptic DAT (which also transports noradrenaline), this does not seem to be the full picture and methylphenidate appears to reverse the action of the DAT across the cell membrane, causing massive catecholamine neurotransmitter efflux from the neuron into the synapse. In this respect its action is ultimately rather similar to that of dexamfetamine.

Dexamfetamine
[This spelling, with an *f*, is now the official spelling in Europe as the recommended international non-proprietary name (rINN). The more familiar spelling: *dexamphetamine*, although still widely used, is out of date. In the USA it is *dextroamphetamine*.]

Dexamfetamine is the d-isomer of amfetamine, the l-isomer being considerably less potent, although longer lasting. The actions of both isomers of amfetamine are quite complex. It has been known for years that it blocks noradrenaline reuptake from the noradrenergic synapse by competitive substrate blockade of the noradrenaline transporter on the presynaptic neuron membrane. Because monoamine transporters are fairly non-specific ('promiscuous' in technical terms) and in this instance the noradrenaline transporter can also take up dopamine, this means amfetamine will also block dopamine reuptake by the same transporter, albeit rather weakly.

This is important in the prefrontal cortex where there are relatively few DAT sites at neuronal synapses but plenty of noradrenaline transporter sites. The noradrenaline transporters there become flooded by extracellular dopamine and ordinarily take this up too. When amfetamine acts as a noradrenaline transporter blocker in the cortex, it also inhibits dopamine reuptake by the noradrenaline transporter so that both neurotransmitters become more plentiful in the synaptic cleft.

In addition to this (Heal et al. 2013), there is intraneuronal release of monoamines. As the reuptake blocking action is a competitive one, amfetamine itself hijacks the transporter and is thus taken into the neuron cytoplasm, an action different from that of methylphenidate's simple blockade of the membrane transporter. Once inside the neuron, amfetamine is further absorbed by the vesicular monoamine transporter (VMAT2), which transfers newly created or reabsorbed monoamines from the cytoplasm into vesicles for storage. This means that amfetamine is actively transported into these vesicles and so displaces large amounts of monoamines (noradrenaline and dopamine) into the neuronal cytoplasm, something that then opens cell membrane channels, releasing monoamines into the synaptic cleft. It can also reverse the action of the reuptake transporter at the cell membrane so that dopamine and noradrenaline in a ratio of roughly 4:1 are rapidly pumped into the cleft. Unlike the action of methylphenidate, there is also a release of a small amount of 5-HT.

This monoamine release within the neuron and the reversal of membrane transport has a considerably greater and more immediate effect than that produced by a selective noradrenaline reuptake inhibitor such as atomoxetine that simply exerts its effect at the neuronal surface.

Stimulant effects on neuropsychological test results

Abnormal neuropsychological findings on a variety of tests and procedures can be identified in ADHD (Swanson et al. 2011). However, there is, as yet, no single test or variable on which stimulants (or any other ADHD medication) have an effect that indicates precisely how they exert their beneficial effect on behaviour. Generally speaking, tests that tap cognitive executive function reflect the ability to inhibit responses, reveal aspects of working memory, or increase motivation in relation to reward, and have been the most profitable areas of scientific enquiry, but we are, as yet, no closer to identifying single testable key areas of neurocognitive function that change in relation to stimulant medication in a manner that would explain the observable change in behaviour.

There is, therefore, no point in obtaining a neuropsychological test baseline against which to titrate medication (Bolea-Alamanac et al. 2014).

Clinical effects

At a clinical level, stimulants promote concentration, increase focus on salient features, promote resistance to distraction and enhance persistence at tasks requiring analytic thought. Certainly they will correct the inattention and disorganisation listed among the features of ADHD, but they go further than that, something parents welcome (Coletti et al. 2012).

Stimulants are cognitive enhancers and their positive effect on a variety of higher cognitive processes, particularly those termed cognitive executive function, goes beyond their alleviation of the deficits and immaturities seen in ADHD. This is evident in real life as far as parental report on the BRIEF behavioural questionnaire (which is held to reflect cognitive executive function) goes (Findling et al. 2013).

Stimulants can enhance working memory in a real-life setting. Laboratory studies show enhancement of spatial rather than the more relevant auditory working memory, but in real-life settings, auditory working memory can also be seen to improve, possibly because of increased motivation for the listening task.

In the medium term, stimulant medications will improve academic functioning when this is directly linked to the child's improved ability to allocate mental effort, sustain learning tasks ranging from learning spelling to revision, or complete longer assignments. They can lead to better examination results if the individual can use planning, time judgement, clearer handwriting and better concentration across a long time period.

On the other hand, they will not have a direct beneficial effect on the literacy difficulties of dyslexia, although they may well enable greater participation in remedial learning activities. Stimulants will also not increase IQ or straightforward short-term memory.

Some of the older children can be emphatic that the medication produces greater clarity of thought or makes it easier for them to concentrate and resist distraction. It is helpful to ask, at review, not just 'Is this medicine working for you?' but also 'How can you tell?'

The effect on mood can be striking. Stimulant medication can assist emotional regulation, especially anger and consequent acute aggressive outbursts. It can reduce a feeling, or manifestation, of excitability. Children may then say that this is accompanied by a subjective feeling of greater 'calmness'. Older teenagers will talk about a lessening of emotional reactions to minor setbacks or triumphs during the day, as is well documented in adult practice. Although increased anxiety can occasionally be seen as an unwanted effect, a reduction of anxiety symptoms is perhaps equally common.

A lessening of irritability is often accompanied by a greater willingness to comply with family or school demands. In clinical terms there can be a diminution of the symptoms of the oppositional-defiant behaviour pattern. Overall, parents are likely to use phrases like 'easier to live with'.

Hyperactivity is calmed without sedation and what becomes evident is better regulation of activity and a reduced feeling of restlessness. The same is true of impulsiveness, and older children will describe how it is simply 'easier' to inhibit impulsive actions and tolerate waiting once the clinician has found the right examples and vocabulary to talk about it with them.

It is often noted that stimulant medication will improve handwriting, and closer examination of this often reveals an improvement in general motor coordination when this coexists (as it often does), so this is not just a reflection of a reduced habit of rushing at a task. Illegal diversion of prescribed stimulants into competitive sport to improve coordination and sometimes stamina is becoming a wider concern.

It is not always necessary to have ADHD to benefit from stimulant medication. These enhancements can be seen in individuals without ADHD, thus improved mental functioning with stimulants is not an indication that the individual has ADHD. There is current concern about the diversion of prescribed stimulants into senior school and college student populations, not for recreational use, but to improve concentration in revision and exams.

Adverse effects

In general terms, the beneficial effects of stimulants increase with dose and it is no longer thought that there is an optimal dose beyond which there is a lessening of cognitive benefit, until it is evident that an excessive dose of stimulant medication has resulted in excessively quiet social withdrawal, loss of facial expression of emotion, and repetitive or perseverative behaviours. At this point it also becomes evident that there is cognitive overfocusing.

There is little difference in adverse effects between methylphenidate and dexamfetamine, although there are differences in individuals' tolerance.

Overall, appetite suppression, perhaps with consequent slowing of weight gain (or even weight loss) is very common. Parents will usually work out ways in which it is possible to provide sufficient food at breakfast and in the evening, although occasionally, especially with the longer sustained-release preparations and lisdexamfetamine, appetite may return late in the evening and interfere with going to bed or settling to sleep. Advice around healthy but high-calorie input at the time of starting medication is valuable. Conversely, the question 'Are you hungry at lunchtime?' is often a subtle way for the clinician to pick up non-adherence, particularly with sustained-release preparations.

Growth issues are discussed in Chapter 8, but in my experience severe difficulties are rare, provided there is close supervision and appropriate advice.

Onset insomnia is a common problem with immediate-release preparations given in the early evening or with some sustained release preparations. In some ways this is not so much a side effect as a primary effect, as both stimulants were originally used to promote wakeful alertness: amfetamine as the 'wakey-wakey' tablets for wartime aircrew, methylphenidate for jaded fatigue in civilians. At weekends and in school holidays, adolescents tend to lie in, so their 'breakfast' medication is taken late and this can then shift their sleep onset time later. In students living away from home this can quite quickly lead to a reversal of day/night activity. Difficulties with falling or staying asleep are common in ADHD and not necessarily medication-related, so this is important to document at an initial assessment. It is very unlikely indeed that waking early is a stimulant effect.

A small and not clinically relevant increase in pulse rate and systolic blood pressure is common, although not inevitable. Monitoring is, however, important to pick up the few outliers. On direct questioning, a number of teenagers will say they sometimes experience bursts of rapid palpitations.

Rebound effects, usually with immediate-release preparations, can occur about an hour or so after a dose has worn off. Excitability, irritability, restlessness and talkativeness can be quite alarming to parents after a first dose of a medication trial unless they are warned of the possibility. A more gradual onset of dysphoria and generally apparent low mood that persists can sometimes be alleviated by a switch to a different stimulant or atomoxetine. Management of these adverse affects by and large follows common sense and is dealt with in the following chapters and in Graham et al. (2011).

Quite a few adolescents complain that methylphenidate in particular constrains their social spontaneity. This is more than their friends finding them less amusing because their impulsiveness no longer irritates teachers; it is a mildly unpleasant subjective sense of feeling inhibited and not socially engaged with one's peers. They may not experience the same effect following a switch to (lis)dexamfetamine.

Less frequent complaints are abdominal pain, headache, increased anxiety, irritability and excited talkativeness. A very few young people have commented to me that they experience a very mild sense of well-being, particularly with dexamfetamine. Usually, tics are not exacerbated, although very occasionally this occurs. The phasic nature of tics means that this is often by coincidence (Friedland & Walkup 2015), and indeed it tends to settle after several weeks. Rather surprisingly, adolescents occasionally complain of loss of stamina in sporting activities, although sustained energy is a more usual finding, perhaps through a motivational effect.

The list of possible, yet rare, adverse effects is long, with hair loss, Raynaud's phenomenon, facial flushing, sensitivity rash, dystonias and auditory hallucinations being worthy of note. Sometimes these appear to be dose-dependent or resolve when a switch is made to the other stimulant.

Although patient information leaflets list a large number of possible side effects about which clinicians should be aware, I have never seen dependency, psychosis (although I have seen children who experience auditory hallucinations), sustained leucopenia or exacerbation of seizure frequency in 40 years of prescribing stimulants for ADHD in childhood.

Parental report or spontaneous complaint is the usual way in which an adverse effect is detected, but this will not always be enough, especially with a monosyllabic adolescent brought unwillingly to clinic. Cox et al. (2015) provided a very useful self-completed questionnaire about both negative and positive side effects.

One additional possible adverse consequence of stimulants is trouble with school or university authorities or the police for sharing or selling them to others. Recreational abuse by snorting immediate-release preparations goes in and out of fashion, and there are requests from friends for pills to help with revision for exams or to help stay awake on long drives or at parties. It is wise to anticipate that this will happen, especially in shared accommodation at university, and advise accordingly (keep quiet about your medication, take it in secret, never give or sell to others).

Long-term use of stimulant medications

It is well known that the long-term follow-ups of the Multimodal Treatment of ADHD study (MTA Study Group 1999) revealed that after three years those children allocated to the intensive medication treatment groups were no longer doing better than those who received the 'community' and psychosocial interventions, in spite of their improved response at 14 months (Jensen et al. 2007; Molina et al. 2009). This is, however, difficult to interpret, as the treatment groups were not kept distinct after 14 months, so there was the possibility of those from the intensive medication arm stopping their treatment and those in the behavioural arm commencing medication. Discussion of the interpretation of long-term MTA data continues (Hinshaw et al. 2015). Generally speaking, the MTA children were milder cases than would probably be seen in UK services (Santosh et al. 2005) and thus more likely to mature out of their diagnosis during follow-up.

The loss of effect over time has not been confirmed in other studies (Swanson et al. 2011). Clinical experience and a number of studies show that children and young people can continue to benefit for several years (Harpin et al. 2016), although there will be attrition because of lessening adherence to medication and some will no longer need medication following symptom improvement with maturation.

It is intriguing that the sample of young adolescents who continued to take medication for their ADHD over a 4-year period showed a smaller decrease in frontal cerebral cortex thickness, approximating to normal developmental change, than those who did not (Shaw et al. 2009). There are similar findings with respect to normalisation of grey matter development in the basal ganglia in medicated compared with non-medicated children (Nakao & Radua 2011).

Preparations

Methylphenidate

Other than a patch version (not available in Europe) that uses a transdermal drug delivery system, all stimulant preparations are orally administered. Typically, the behavioural effects are seen within 30 to 60 minutes after swallowing.

Tablets and capsules are the usual form of administration, although a 5mg/5ml liquid is available to special order in the UK. The ordinary immediate-release tablets of methylphenidate produce a clinical effect that closely follows the blood level pK (pharmacokinetic) curve and lasts around 3 hours for the basic immediate-release preparation. Accordingly, sustained-release preparations have been developed in order to simplify dosing schedules, increase adherence and reduce the stigma of being observed to take medication (e.g. at school). For methylphenidate, these include capsules with two types of bead, one immediate release, one delayed.

In the USA, an older method for obtaining sustained release is to embed methylphenidate in a methylcellulose matrix, a water-soluble preparation with sustained-release properties.

The OROS methylphenidate system is a considerably more complex mechanism and involves a biphasic or what is effectively a triphasic release with an outer layer of medication coating providing the first phase, supplemented subsequently by osmotic absorption of water, which pumps out active methylphenidate in two waves of increasing concentration from an insoluble capsule.

Methylphenidate is metabolised very rapidly in the liver, and parents are usually gratified to learn that it is ordinarily cleared from the body within the day on which it was given. A small number of children appear to experience enzyme induction and acquire tolerance in the first few months, thus requiring an increase in the daily dose. The need for a further increase of dose in subsequent months does not, in my experience, recur, although over the longer term, higher doses may well be needed as work demands or body mass increase.

Dexamfetamine

Dexamfetamine is available in four forms. In most countries it is most widely available from manufacturers as tablets. In North America, there is a sustained-release capsule form, and a liquid form has recently been released in the UK.

Mixed amfetamine salts (MAS) are a well-known preparation of d-amfetamine and l-amfetamine in 3:1 proportions. They use a sustained-release form using two types of bead to provide an effect lasting 8 hours or longer. This is not easily available in Europe.

A racemic amfetamine with equal amounts of l- and d-isomers exploits the l-isomer's longer time to metabolise so that the effect is still superior to placebo 10 hours after a single dose.

Lisdexamfetamine methylate is an inert prodrug. This covalent compound of dexamfetamine and lysine has no psychoactive properties until absorbed into the bloodstream, where hydrolysis by red blood cells releases active dexamfetamine in a steady rate-limited process that enables it to exert its effects for over 12 hours or longer.

Stimulant preparations are also compared in Appendix 5 (courtesy of Professor Steve Bazire).

Non-stimulant medications

Catecholamine reuptake inhibitors
Atomoxetine
Atomoxetine is currently the most prevalent of the non-stimulant medications effective in the management of ADHD and is available widely internationally as a non-controlled drug with no predilection for abuse. All guidelines suggest atomoxetine may be preferred to stimulants when there is

• comorbid anxiety

• severe tics

• drug abuse in the young person or family

although none of these is an absolute contraindication to stimulants. It should also be considered when 'round the clock' control is essential. Atomoxetine is available in a range of capsules and as an oral solution.

Pharmacology: Atomoxetine is a highly selective noradrenaline reuptake inhibitor active in the prefrontal cortex. The reuptake transporters are not very selective, however, and because the DAT density in the prefrontal cortex is low, there is only slow clearance of dopamine and much dopamine is in fact taken up into noradrenergic neurons by the noradrenaline transporter. Blockade of this transporter thus creates an increase in both noradrenaline and dopamine in the prefrontal cortex, but does not increase dopamine in the striatum where there is a high intensity of DAT sites and effective clearance of extracellular dopamine. Nevertheless, atomoxetine is effective for both inattention and hyperactive/impulsive symptoms.

Dosing: There is an effective dose range from 1.2 to 1.8mg/kg/day. Unlike the stimulants, atomoxetine has a dose beyond which further increase yields no added effect. For most individuals this is around 1.8mg/kg/day.

Although the manufacturer recommends morning dosing, there is no reason not to take it in the evening, and this may lead to better tolerance of the possible side effects of drowsiness or persisting nausea or abdominal pain.

There is variation in how rapidly atomoxetine is metabolised by the liver (via the cytochrome P450 enzyme pathway). About 10% of people are 'slow metabolisers' and they are somewhat more prone to adverse effects. Although it is technically possible to identify whether someone is a slow metaboliser ahead of time, this is cumbersome, so it makes more sense simply to bear the possibility in mind and monitor progress. Similarly, a few children, considered to be fast metabolisers, do better on twice-daily dosing.

Main effect: The main clinical effect of atomoxetine is to improve the clinical symptoms of ADHD in a manner that is qualitatively the same as stimulants. Occasional studies have indicated a small positive effect on anxiety and low mood, but this is not consistent, and low mood may present as an unwanted effect. Atomoxetine does not inhibit sleep onset in the way that stimulants can.

Since its release in 2002 in the USA and in 2004 in Europe, there has been an evolving understanding of the clinical course of improvement with atomoxetine, and a number of misunderstandings need correction (Bushe & Savill 2011). Although atomoxetine's action as a reuptake inhibitor is potent, it has been held that its clinical efficacy is moderate. An effect size of 0.6 is widely quoted. In fact, the effect size increases with time, and at 12 weeks is 0.8 and still rising (Montoya et al. 2009). An even higher effect size of 1.3 was found in one study after 10 weeks when combined with psychoeducation (Svanborg et al. 2009).

In terms of the proportion of responders, Wang and colleagues (2007) found atomoxetine not to be inferior to methylphenidate in that about 80% of children responded to each. In a 6-week comparison trial with OROS methylphenidate, Newcorn et al. (2008) found that, of the individuals who did not respond to methylphenidate, 43% subsequently responded to atomoxetine. Similarly, 42% of those who did not respond to atomoxetine responded to methylphenidate. Oddly, admission to the trial excluded previous non-responders to methylphenidate, which would bias the figures.

Side effects: Minor side effects are well recognised. Nausea, perhaps vomiting, is moderately prevalent in the first day or two of taking it. The risk is lessened by starting slowly and by ensuring medication is given after a meal.

Appetite suppression is common but tends to be less emphatic than can be the case with stimulants. Slowing of weight and height growth can occur, but returns to previous growth trajectories after 42 months (Spencer et al. 2007). Persisting nausea, drowsiness and irritability are not uncommon, and older adolescents may complain of sexual dysfunction.

The effects on the cardiovascular system are closely comparable to those of the stimulants: a rise in pulse rate of about 10bpm is common, as is a slight rise in blood pressure (4mmHg). In 6–12% of children this can be greater and sometimes increase progressively (MHRA 2012), so atomoxetine would be contraindicated in children with some cardiovascular or cerebrovascular conditions, and blood pressure should always be monitored. The blood pressure tables published by Great Ormond Street Hospital for Children (http://www.gosh.nhs.uk/health-professionals/clinical-guidelines/blood-pressure-monitoring#Appendices) are recommended, because they display a 95% limit in line with MHRA guidance.

An early concern about possible risk of liver injury following atomoxetine has abated, and the risk is now considered minimal or absent (e.g. Bangs et al. 2008). There is no value in regular liver function tests.

There have been a few reports of psychotic or manic symptoms at conventional therapeutic doses in individuals with no prior history of these (MHRA 2009). Whether this differs from the risk with stimulants is not known.

Although regulatory authorities in both the UK and the USA have issued warnings that treatment with atomoxetine is associated with a small increase in suicidal ideation (0.37% (5/1357) in Bangs et al. 2008) over placebo in clinical trials, there have been no actual suicides. There were also doubts as to whether the rates for suicidal ideation or suicidal behaviour rate in patients taking atomoxetine were raised compared with methylphenidate. Bushe and Savill (2013), in a meta-analysis, found no difference between the two treatments and, most recently, Chen et al. (2014) in a large register study found no increase in actual suicidal behaviour associated with any ADHD medication (including atomoxetine). Indeed, they conclude that their findings suggested a protective effect from treatment, perhaps by reducing impulsivity. Overall, it seems plausible that there is a slight rise in the rate of suicidal ideation associated with medication, but this is not translated into suicidal behaviour.

Indications: The patient or their family may prefer atomoxetine for convenience, because it is not a controlled drug and its protracted effect means it can usually be taken once daily with benefits extending effectively for 24 hours in most people.

It is possible to combine atomoxetine and methylphenidate in order to extend treatment across the full day (off licence). The rate of side effects increases, however. There is no point combining it with dexamfetamine as both act predominantly on the noradrenaline transporter.

Clonidine and guanfacine

α_2-Adrenoceptor agonists

These include *clonidine* and *guanfacine*. Neither are controlled drugs. Clonidine is approved for ADHD treatment in its extended-release form in the USA, but not in the UK. Guanfacine has an extended-release preparation (guanfacine XR in the scientific literature, where the XR tag indicates a sustained-release form using two types of bead to provide an effect lasting 8 hours or longer). This is available as an immediate-release preparation in the USA.

Main effect: Both clonidine and guanfacine are α2-receptor adrenergic agonists. Clonidine acts on all adrenergic α_2-receptors (α_2a-, α_2b- and α_2c-receptors) present in the prefrontal cortex, thalamus and locus coeruleus, but guanfacine is more selective for the α_2a-receptors and is thus less likely to produce some of the common side effects of immediate-release clonidine.

Immediate-release guanfacine has a very short half-life in children (although not in adults) so guanfacine only became a viable ADHD treatment once the sustained-release form was developed.

In the prefrontal cortex the agonistic action enhances noradrenergic signalling by action on the α_2-receptors on the axonal surface of the postsynaptic neurones of the prefrontal cortex. The result is an improved signal-to-noise ratio in neuronal transmission. In addition, there appears to be an important positive effect of guanfacine on the dendritic spines of the pyramidal neurones of layer III of the dorso-lateral prefrontal cortex, the site of working memory. There is a direct promotion of dendritic spine growth and activity, so microcircuits in that layer can maintain firing after a visual or auditory perceptual stimulus, enable short-term and working memory, and thus strengthen cognitive control of behaviour and facilitate resisting impulsiveness or distraction (Arnsten & Jin 2012).

The potency of adrenergic α_2-receptors in treating ADHD is less than that of stimulants, with an effect size of about 0.6–0.9 depending on the variable measured (Biederman et al. 2008; Hervas et al. 2014).

Indications: The usefulness of α_2-receptor agonists rests partly on their ability to provide 24-hour cover for ADHD symptoms. Guanfacine XR can be given daily as a single dose at any time of day. Another potential aspect of their usefulness is their reported ability to lessen tic activity and reduce aggressive behaviour.

Side effects: Although side effects are rather more evident for clonidine, in both medications sedation somnolence and fatigue (SSF) are common. For guanfacine XR this tends to wear off after about 3 weeks. Both can cause a slight lowering of blood pressure and slowing of pulse rate. Dry mouth, constipation and intolerance of cold weather are seen mainly with clonidine. Generally speaking, they do not affect appetite, although there are some reports of weight gain with guanfacine XR. Some of this is probably because trial participants have gained weight after discontinuing stimulants just before entering the trial.

Clonidine can be given in immediate-release form at night to counteract onset insomnia. This does not seem to occur with guanfacine XR, where a steady state is reached.

In spite of concerns 20 years ago, it is now accepted that it is safe to combine an α_2-receptor agonist with a stimulant. An obvious role for either drug would be to supplement and complement stimulant medication, although the current European regulatory approval is for solo use. As clonidine and guanfacine (Scahill et al. 2001) can be beneficial in tic disorders, they have a theoretical use as an alternative to stimulants or to be co-prescribed with them for children who have ADHD with tics.

Other preparations
Bupropion
Bupropion was originally developed as an antidepressant and is also used as an aid to giving up smoking. It is not approved for use by the under-18s but is occasionally used off-label for ADHD.

There is some uncertainty as to its pharmacological action, although Heal et al. (2011) argue that it is probably both a noradrenaline and dopamine reuptake inhibitor, confirming the unreferenced description by Stahl and Mignon (2011). It produces only a moderate improvement in ADHD symptoms in adults, and the National Institute for

Health and Care Excellence (NICE 2008) was unimpressed by the evidence for use in children.

The clumsy dosing in the only form available in the UK limits its use. A history of seizures is an absolute contraindication.

Modafinil

The indication for modafinil as a treatment for narcolepsy or other causes of sleepiness, and the fact that it can enhance cognitive functioning, suggests to some that it is in fact effectively a stimulant, but its precise mode of action is unknown. Although only a mild inhibitor of dopamine reuptake *in vitro*, it binds to DATs *in vivo* and produces a slow, modest efflux of dopamine, noradrenaline and serotonin in both prefrontal cortex and striatum (Heal et al. 2011). In most countries, although not in the UK, it is a controlled drug.

It produces an improvement in ADHD symptoms and would probably have been approved for the treatment of ADHD in childhood were it not for a single treatment emergent case of apparent Stevens–Johnson syndrome in trials. It is used off-label with some success, and NICE (2008) considered the evidence for its effect in ADHD to be positive. Its side effects are generally similar to those of stimulants.

Tricyclic antidepressants

For many years, imipramine, nortriptyline, amitriptyline and desipramine were the only available non-stimulant treatments for ADHD. They are all monoamine reuptake inhibitors, binding predominantly with the noradrenaline transporter, with varying degrees of selectivity. They had only a moderate effect on ADHD symptoms, mainly on hyperactivity, which not uncommonly wore off after several months.

Mounting concern about cardiac side effects (particularly following a few deaths with desipramine) and their high toxicity in overdose led them to be largely abandoned as treatments for ADHD after the release of atomoxetine, although they are used very occasionally when there is no viable alternative.

Summary

- Medication for ADHD is generally classified into stimulants and non-stimulants, and in most instances children start with a trial of a stimulant, most commonly methylphenidate.

- About one-quarter of all children will respond better to one stimulant than the other, so a poor response to an initial stimulant should lead promptly to trial with the other. This can lead to very high rates of positive response.

- Stimulants work by catecholamine reuptake blockade coupled with release of catecholamines into the synaptic cleft.

- Extended-release formulations of stimulants follow a range of principles: e.g. wax-coated beads, OROS release system, enzymatic lysis of a prodrug within the bloodstream.

- Appetite suppression and onset insomnia are common adverse effects of stimulants, as are a small increase in pulse rate and blood pressure.

- Long-term prescription of stimulants appears to have beneficial effects on brain growth and development.

- Non-stimulants have different modes of action. In particular, atomoxetine is a pure noradrenaline reuptake inhibitor and guanfacine mimics the effect of noradrenaline on post-synaptic neuron receptors.

- Non-stimulants have somewhat smaller effect sizes than stimulants, but can have an effect over a full 24 hours.

- The choice of non-stimulant over stimulant is often driven by an attempt to minimise side effects.

- Atomoxetine takes weeks to achieve optimal effect.

- The risk of suicidal behaviour associated with atomoxetine has probably been overstated.

- Prolonged-release guanfacine may be particularly useful in children with both ADHD and tic disorders.

- All licensed medications for ADHD in the UK, with the exception of guanfacine, are now available in liquid or soluble form.

References

Arnold LE (2000) Methylphenidate vs amphetamine: Comparative review. *J Atten Disord* 3: 200–211, doi:10.1177/108705470000300403.

Arnsten A, Jin L (2012) Guanfacine for the treatment of cognitive disorders: A century of discoveries at Yale. *Yale J Biol Med* 85: 45–58.

Bangs M, Tauscher-Wisniewski S, Polzer J et al (2008) Meta-analysis of suicide-related behaviour events in patients treated with atomoxetine. *J Am Acad Child Adolesc Psychiatry* 47: 209–218, doi:10.1097/chi.0b013e31815d88b2.

Biederman J, Melmed R, Patel A et al. (2008) A randomized, double-blind, placebo-controlled study of guanfacine extended release in children and adolescents with attention-deficit/hyperactivity disorder. *Pediatrics* 121: e73–e84.

Bolea-Alamanac B, Nutt D, Adamou M et al. (2014) Evidence-based guidelines for the pharmacological management of attention deficit hyperactivity disorder: Update on recommendations from the British Association for Psychopharmacology. *J Psychopharmacol* 28: 179–203, doi:10.1177/0269881113519509.

Bushe C, Savill N (2011) Atomoxetine in children and adolescents with attention-deficit/hyperactivity disorder. Systematic review of review papers 2009–2011. An update for clinicians. *J Cent Nerv Syst Dis* 3: 209–217, doi:10.4137/JCNSD.S4391.

Bushe C, Savill N (2013) Suicide related events and attention deficit hyperactivity disorder: A meta-analysis of atomoxetine and methylphenidate comparator clinical trials. *Child Adolesc Psychiatry Mental Health* 7: 19.

Chen Q, Sjolander A, Runeson B et al. (2014) Drug treatment for attention-deficit/hyperactivity disorder and suicidal behaviour: Register based study. *BMJ* 348: g3769, doi:10.1136/bmj.g3769.

Coletti D, Pappadopulos E, Katsiotas N et al. (2012) Parent perspectives on the decision to initiate medication treatment of attention-deficit/hyperactivity disorder. *J Child Adolesc Psychopharm* 22: 226–237, doi:10.1089/cap.2011.0090.

Cox DJ, Davis, MT, Cox BS et al. (2015) Quantifying the relationship between perceived consequences of ADHD medication and its usage. *J Attent Disord* 19: 78–83, doi:10.1177/1087054712452913.

Findling R, Adeyi B, Dirks B et al. (2013) Parent-reported executive function behaviors and clinician ratings of attention-deficit/hyperactivity disorder symptoms in children treated with lisdexamfetamine dimesylate. *J Child Adolesc Psychopharm* 23: 28–35, doi:10.1089/cap.2011.0120.

Friedland S, Walkup J (2015) Meta-assurance: No tic exacerbation caused by stimulants. *J Am Acad Child Adolesc Psychiatry* 54: 706–708, doi:10.1016/j.jaac.2015.06.018.

Graham J, Banaschewski T, Buitelaar J et al. (2011) European guidelines on managing adverse effects of medication for ADHD. *Eur Child Adolesc Psychiatry* 20: 17–37, doi:10.1007/s00787-010-0140-6.

Harpin V, Mazzone L, Raynaud JP, Kahle J, Hodgkins P (2016) Long-term outcomes of ADHD: A systematic review of self-esteem and social function. *J Attent Disord* 20: 295–305.

Heal DJ, Smith SL, Gosden J, Nutt DJ (2013) Amphetamine past and present – a pharmacological and clinical perscive. *J Psychopharmacol* 6: 479–496, doi:10.1177/0269881113482532.

Heal DJ, Smith SL, Findling RL (2011) ADHD: Current and future therapeutics. In: Stanford C, Tannock R, eds. *Behavioral neuroscience of attention deficit hyperactivity disorder and its treatment*, Current Topics in Behavioral Neurosciences 9. Berlin, Heidelberg: Springer.

Hervas A, Huss M, Johnson M, Robertson B (2014) Efficacy and safety of extended-release guanfacine hydrochloride in children and adolescents with attention-deficit/hyperactivity disorder: A randomized, controlled, phase III trial. *Eur Neuropsychopharmacol* 24: 1861–1872, doi:10.1007/7584_2011_125.

Hinshaw SP, Arnold LE and the MTA Cooperative Group (2015) Attention-deficit hyperactivity disorder, multimodal treatment, and longitudinal outcome: evidence, paradox, and challenge. *Wiley Interdiscip Rev Cogn Sci* 6(1): 39–52, doi:10.1002/wcs.1324.

Hodgkins P, Shaw M, Coghill D, Hechtman L (2012) Amfetamine and methylphenidate medications for attention-deficit disorder: Complementary treatment options. *Eur Child Adolesc Psychiatry* 21: 477–492, doi:10.1007/s00787-012-0286-5.

Holden SE, Jenkins Jones S, Poole C et al. (2013) The prevalence and incidence, resource use and financial costs of treating people with attention deficit/hyperactivity disorder (ADHD) in the United Kingdom (1998 to 2010). *Child Adolesc Psychiatry Mental Health* 7: 34, doi:10.1186/1753-2000-7-34.

Jensen PS, Arnold LE, Swanson JM et al. (2007) Three-year follow-up of the NIMH MTA study. *J Am Acad Child Adolesc Psychiatry* 46(8): 989–1002.

MHRA (Medical and Healthcare Products Regulatory Agency) (2009) Atomoxetine: risk of psychotic or manic symptoms in children and adolescents; available at https://www.gov.uk/drug-safety-update/atomoxetine-risk-of-psychotic-or-manic-symptoms-in-children-and-adolescents.

MHRA (2012) Atomoxetine (Strattera): increases in blood pressure and heart rate; available at https://www.gov.uk/drug-safety-update/atomoxetine-strattera-increases-in-blood-pressure-and-heart-rate.

Molina BS, Hinshaw SP, Swanson JM et al., MTA Cooperative Group (2009) The MTA at 8 years: prospective follow-up of children treated for combined-type ADHD in a multisite study. *J Am Acad Child Adolesc Psychiatry* 48(5): 484–500, doi:10.1097/CHI.0b013e31819c23d0.

Montoya A, Hervas A, Cardo E et al. (2009) Evaluation of atomoxetine for first-line treatment of newly diagnosed, treatment-naïve children and adolescents with attention deficit/hyperactivity disorder. *Curr Med Res Opin* 25: 2745–2754, doi:10.1185/03007990903316152.

MTA Study Group (1999) A 14-month randomized clinical trial of treatment strategies for attention-deficit/hyperactivity disorder. The MTA Cooperative Group. Multimodal Treatment Study of Children with ADHD. *Arch Gen Psychiatry* 56(12): 1073–1086.

Nakao T, Radua J (2011) Gray matter volume abnormalities in ADHD and the effects of stimulant medication: Voxel-based meta-analysis. *Am J Psychiatry* 168: 1154–1163.

Newcorn JH, Kratochvil CJ, Allen AJ et al. (2008) Atomoxetine and osmotically released methylphenidate for the treatment of attention deficit hyperactivity disorder: acute comparison and differential response. *Am J Psychiatry* 165: 721–730, doi:10.1176/appi.ajp.2007.05091676.

NICE (2008) *Attention deficit hyperactivity disorder: Diagnosis and management. NICE Clinical Guidelines* [CG72], https://www.nice.org.uk/guidance/cg72.

Ramtvedt BE, Røinas E, Aabach HS, Sundet KS (2013) Clinical gains from including both dextroamphetamine and methylphenidate in stimulant trials. *J Child Adolesc Psychopharmacol* 23: 597–604, doi:10.1089/cap.2012.0085.

Santosh PJ, Taylor E, Swanson J et al. (2005) Refining the diagnoses of inattention and overactivity syndromes: A reanalysis of the Multimodal Treatment Study of attention-deficit hyperactivity disorder (ADHD) based on ICD-10 criteria for hyperkinetic disorder. *Clin Neurosci Res* 5: 307–314, doi:10.1016/j.cnr.2005.09.010.

Scahill L, Chappell P, Kim Y et al. (2001) A placebo-controlled study of guanfacine in the treatment of children with tic disorders and attention deficit hyperactivity disorder. *Am J Psychiatry* 158(7): 1067–1074, doi:10.1176/appi.ajp.158.7.1067.

Shaw P, Sharp W, Morrison M et al. (2009) Psychostimulant treatment and the developing cortex in attention deficit hyperactivity disorder. *Am J Psychiatry* 166: 56–63.

Spencer T, Kratochvil C, Sangal B et al. (2007) Effects of atomoxetine on growth in children with attention-deficit/hyperactivity disorder following up to five years of treatment. *J Child Adolesc Psychopharmacol* 17: 689–699, doi:10.1089/cap.2006.0100.

Stahl SM, Mignon L (2011) *Stahl's illustrated attention deficit hyperactivity disorder.* New York, NY: Cambridge University Press.

Svanborg P, Thernlund G, Gustafsson PA et al. (2009) Efficacy and safety of atomoxetine as add-on to psychoeducation in the treatment of attention deficit/hyperactivity disorder: A randomized double-blind, placebo-controlled study in stimulant-naïve Swedish children and adolescents. *Eur Child Adolesc Psychiatry* 18: 240–249, doi:10.1007/s00787-008-0725-5.

Swanson J, Baier RD, Volkow ND (2011) Understanding the effects of stimulant medication on cognition in individuals with attention-deficit hyperactivity disorder: A decade of progress. *Neuropsychopharmacology* 36: 207–226, doi:10.1038/npp.2010.160.

Wang Y, Zheng Y, Du Y et al. (2007) Atomoxetine *versus* methylphenidate in paediatric outpatients with attention deficit hyperactivity disorder: a randomized, double-blind comparison trial. *Aust N Z J Psychiatry* 41: 222–230, doi:10.1080/00048670601057767.

Chapter 7

Using, monitoring and optimising medication

Peter Hill

Dear Dr,

We are writing to express our thoughts regarding Jamie's general behaviour and ability and our difficulties parenting him.

I, Kate, have attended the 10-week ADHD parenting course which was both enlightening and helpful. We are trying to apply some of the behavioural techniques suggested, and use the book '123 Magic'. However life continues to be difficult. Our difficulties include Jamie not listening, or choosing to ignore. This poses a problem when out and about, when Jamie walks off, or takes himself to anything that interests him, not doing anything when asked, for example, in a car park when danger is present. His general confrontation when asked to do anything that does not suit him, and constant use of silly language such as 'idiot' and 'stupid', and hitting/kicking me and his brothers. These seem to be daily challenges.

Tom and I continue to discuss medication and now as time passes on, and Jamie continues to grow and mature, we would be grateful for anything that can make Jamie more likable to others, make life easier for him, and help him reach his potential. However, we are not sure if medication actually helps with the abovementioned confrontational behaviour.

(Letter from parents of a primary-school-age child with ADHD sent to inform discussion about starting medication)

Having considered the currently available medications for the treatment of ADHD in Chapter 6, this chapter will focus on using them in clinical practice. I will assume that the child (a term that includes adolescents) has been fully assessed by a specialist, is at least 6 years old, lives in a family context and attends school. The last three conditions are not of course a requirement for medication, but are assumed here for the sake of simplicity of language. In other settings what is said here may need some modification, usually in an obvious way. There is a later special section on preschool children.

I have adopted a personal tone for some paragraphs as advice on the fine detail of clinical practice is not often dealt with in the scientific literature. What I suggest is not going to be the only way of going about things but it is based on nearly 40 years of practice in ADHD.

All guidelines for childhood ADHD advocate combining medication with non-pharmacological interventions including psychoeducation. Providing information about ADHD, behavioural management and medication is important on common-sense grounds in order to facilitate independence and empowerment and to promote adherence to prescribed medication. When evidence-based information, in lay terms, is provided by the treating clinician it can also balance, counteract or amplify information and misinformation the family will receive from the internet, relatives or newspapers and magazines (sometimes it seems that everyone is an expert on ADHD medication). A good principle is to provide the patient and family at the outset with a handout about medication and details of some reliable sources of information (official guidelines, patient support groups) as well as providing a further small item of information about ADHD or its treatment at every follow-up appointment. Psychoeducation and behavioural management are discussed further in Chapter 5.

Introducing the idea of medication to the child and family

Some families know about medication and want it. Others are set against it. Many are unsure and apprehensive as to whether this is an irreversible, potentially damaging or irresponsible intervention. It often pays to acknowledge mixed or negative attitudes openly, especially when disagreement is likely. Fathers and grandparents who have not attended the clinic may be against the idea, sometimes making medication trials impossible. Once again, providing balanced written information to read and refer to outside the consultation is helpful.

As it is the child or young person who will be taking the medication it is right and proper to include them in the discussion. Personally, I find it useful to make it clear to them that it is me who is prescribing it and it is their medicine, using just that word rather than the word 'drug', which leads children who have had drug-awareness lessons at school to the wrong idea. I explain that it is to help them manage their concentration, to behave more calmly and to help them to stay out of trouble with everyone (or whatever terms arise from the previous assessment). I point out that it usually helps people with ADHD a great deal but that we have to find out whether it suits them. I say that if everyone agrees that it does not suit them or does not work, we can stop it immediately. I also add that I am not going to do anything harmful or dangerous. By talking directly to the child in the presence of the parents, I am informing them too.

It is wise to raise the question of unwanted effects at this point (Gajria et al. 2014), saying that it may mean they are not hungry for lunch, that if they take it too late in the day it will keep them awake. If it gives them a headache or tummy pain or makes them worried ('anxious' is not widely understood by children) then they should say so. Say to parents directly that this medicine is not going to cause addiction or brain damage.

If they ask how it works, point out that we know a great deal about this medicine; it has been around for a long time. It stimulates the front of the brain to work better and boost concentration, control excited hyperactivity and resist the temptation to do something silly or dangerous. Pictures of functional brain scans showing the impact of medication visually often have enormous positive impact.

Recognise that one of the first things parents or older children will do when they get home is go to the internet and look everything up. It makes sense to list websites for organisations (Attention Deficit Disorder Information and Support Service (ADDISS), Children and Adults with Attention-Deficit/Hyperactivity Disorder (CHADD), Canadian ADHD Resource Alliance (CADDRA), etc.) or standard guidelines on a written handout and to point out that there is a great deal of mischievous and wrong information out there. There may well be other children taking medication at the child's school and it is worth asking older children about this and what they think about it.

A common parental fear is that in some way they are embarking on a 'slippery slope' and it is therefore helpful to acknowledge this and say that it is not like that. Everything is done on a step-by-step basis with each step being justified to everyone and with everyone's agreement. Reassure them that the medicine can be stopped at any time if it is not working or if there is concern about its effects.

A further widely shared parental anxiety is that their child will become a 'zombie' or lose his or her personality. It is straightforward to say you are just not going to let that happen and that you will make sure he or she does not receive too high a dose.

If the medicine in question is a controlled drug, explain that this is because some people in the past have used it for themselves illegally and dangerously in very high doses to get high. Say that it is not dangerous in the doses used for the treatment of ADHD and will not make the child become dependent on it or get high. When using non-stimulants, explain that it is not possible to get high at all. Children, young people and adults with ADHD are at increased risk for future substance misuse (mainly nicotine and alcohol but also cannabis and cocaine). It is now thought that when serious antisocial behaviour is associated with ADHD it is this and the risk-taking impulsive behaviour of untreated ADHD that increase the likelihood of substance misuse. Medication does not make future drug abuse more likely and may indeed be protective (Zulauf et al. 2014).

Parents sometimes worry that the child will attribute any improvement to the medicine and not to their own efforts. This is very unlikely (Pelham et al. 1997) and if anything, self-esteem rises with improvement in ADHD symptoms and lessening of impairment.

Setting goals and targets: getting beyond improvement

The big trap in using medication is its effectiveness. Symptoms usually improve with initial dosing, within hours or days with stimulants, and everyone is pleased. The temptation for clinician and family is to relax at that point and consider treatment to be sufficiently successful. However, outcomes can be much more effective if a target is set beforehand and treatment success judged by achievement of that.

At review after starting treatment, being satisfied with 'better' is not enough.

It is vital that the child and family should understand what treatment is ultimately intended to achieve and understand what that means in real terms. In adolescents this is a crucial element in making sure they actually take their medicine. This leads to using a triangle of discussion involving the child/young person, the family and the clinician (Box 7.1), ensuring that everyone's view is taken into account and used to develop a management plan owned by all.

There are two ways of thinking about what treatment may achieve. One is to consider a reduction in the total picture of core ADHD symptoms as indicated by scores on a questionnaire such as the ADHD Rating Scale (ADHD-RS), the Conners Scale or SNAP-IV (Swanson, Nolan and Pelham – IV). In clinical trials, a score reduction of 30–50% has been used as a measure of success, but current thinking is that a reduction to a score equivalent to symptom abolition is more desirable. ADHD-RS or SNAP-IV scoring is 0, 1, 2 and 3 for each ADHD symptom so that, for combined ADHD, a top score (of 3 on each of 18 items) would be 54 and reduction of all symptoms to 0 or 1 would be a maximum of 18. This is a possible target but carries the risk of over-medication and does not include a measurement of impairment. The advantage of using a rating scale is that progress is easily expressed as a score or profile so that information about progress and achievement is clear to all.

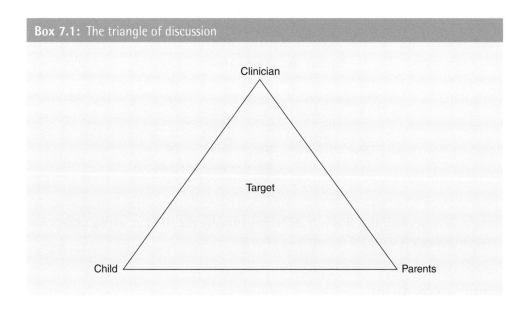

Box 7.1: The triangle of discussion

The second is to identify and agree on a specific treatment goal in which the focus is to reduce a problem arising from the ADHD or impairment associated with it rather than the total symptom count. If the presenting clinical scenario is a child whose ADHD means that suspension from school is imminent or whose family is on the point of fracture because of his behaviour, then the primary aim of treatment may well be to avoid either consequence. If there is less of a crisis there may be features that can be targeted for improvement because they stand out as the reason for referral or family concern. Disruptive behaviour in class, severe personal disorganisation, or an adolescent's inability to revise for exams are examples. For these problems, reliance on a core symptom questionnaire will miss the point, but a target of problem resolution (e.g. no detentions for classroom misbehaviour in a week or completion of revision targets) can be agreed and intermediate steps identified, perhaps on a simple scale, in order to assess progress. The child should be able to understand what the target is, which means it should be in simple behavioural terms and quantified (e.g. 'getting dressed on your own every school-day morning for a week', 'sitting at the table for the whole of mealtime every day for a week'). This can then be translated into a simple scale designed by the child, family and clinician together (for an example see Box 7.2).

One can, in an ideal world, do both and add in a measure of quality of life, although a valid and convenient method for assessing this is still to be developed (Danckaerts et al. 2010). It is generally better to have a structured discussion about the topic, including the child's views, but time pressures on appointments may be a constraint. In this

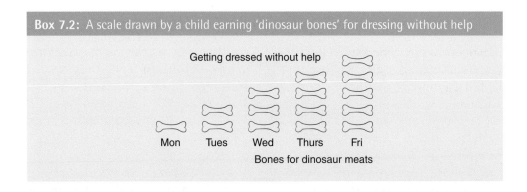

Box 7.2: A scale drawn by a child earning 'dinosaur bones' for dressing without help

Getting dressed without help

Mon   Tues   Wed   Thurs   Fri

Bones for dinosaur meats

context, bear in mind that it is very difficult to involve the child in setting targets and reviewing progress if the follow-up is by phone.

Choice of medicine

Box 7.3 illustrates recommended practice around the choice of medications and when to change from one to another. All current guidelines recommend using methylphenidate as the first-line medication. Although most clinicians do start with methylphenidate, it is important to remember that this is not always going to be the best option. There is roughly a one in four chance that the child is a preferential amfetamine responder and, unless this is borne in mind, there is the risk that the clinician sticks with methylphenidate, fruitlessly substituting one sustained-release preparation for another in an attempt to get a worthwhile response.

Using atomoxetine or an alpha$_2$ (α_2) agonist is another option. It is important to consider atomoxetine or a prolonged-release α_2 agonist used alone if there is concern that a stimulant might intensify tics or anxiety, if there is a risk of stimulant misuse (by any member of the family), or if control across the day to include early mornings or evenings is important.

The impact of ADHD is manifest across the day, sometimes with the most severe difficulties being in the early morning or in the evening. Stimulants have a powerful effect that is seen rapidly after initiation during the day when used alone, but it can be difficult to obtain control at these times, and families may be left to struggle. Currently, combining medications is off licence, but in practice, a combination of a stimulant with an α_2 agonist or sometimes atomoxetine is increasingly used.

Initiating stimulant medication

There are two approaches in general use as far as initiating stimulants are concerned: a single dose trial at home or progressive titration over days and weeks in both home and school (Box 7.4).

Single dose trial at home

One option is to carry out single-dose trials starting with methylphenidate. My practice is to prescribe a small number of 5mg immediate-release methylphenidate tablets. The child is given a 5mg dose at home under a parent's eye one weekend or holiday morning, and 1 hour later is observed doing some settled pencil and paper work simulating classwork or homework. The exercise is repeated on another morning with a 10mg dose, then discussed with the clinician, perhaps by e-mail or phone. This provides an indication of the child's tolerance of methylphenidate and a rough indication of whether it works. If necessary, the exercise can be repeated with single 15 and 20mg doses. It is wise to warn parents that there may occasionally be a phase of irritability in the afternoon as the methylphenidate wears off.

Box 7.3: Recommended practice when medication is indicated

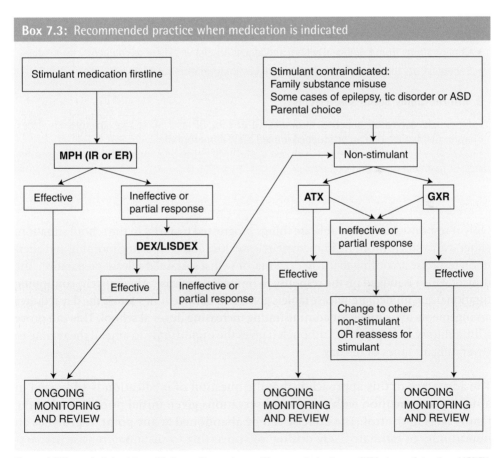

Notes: MPH, methylphenidate; IR, immediate release; ER, extended release; DEX, dexamfetamine; LISDEX: lisdexamfetamine; ASD, autism spectrum disorder; ATX, atomoxetine; XR, guanfacine extended (prolonged) release.

Box 7.4: Initiating methylphenidate: two strategies

1. Single dose trial at home at weekend or in holidays

- Test effect of immediate release (IR) methylphenidate, 5mg, then 10mg, perhaps 15mg

or

- Sustained release preparation 5mg, then 10mg, 20mg etc. or 18mg, 27mg, 36mg
- Will need good communication with parent (phone, email, text) to discuss titration
- Once IR dose seems OK, convert to sustained release, pro-rating dose
- Benefits: Quick result. Puts parents in control and stepwise process is reassuring

2. Progressive titration of whole regime across day

- Immediate release twice or (better) three times daily

or

- Sustained release of choice daily
- Obtain ratings from home and school and adjust dose(s) weekly or as frequently as possible
- Benefits: Cuts the corner of single dose trial estimation of required dose.

3. Inform family about side effects

For example decreased appetite, insomnia, GI effects, BP and pulse rate changes etc. (see Chapter 6). Medication can be stopped immediately if appropriate.

Notes: GI, gastrointestinal; BP, blood pressure.

Only if responses are favourable are things progressed to a trial in the school situation, either with a single morning immediate-release dose and contrasting morning and afternoon response according to teacher reports, or with a sustained-release preparation, the dose of which is judged on the response to immediate-release. Alternatively, continuing titration using immediate-release tablets given two or three times across the day requires arrangements to be made for administrating increasing doses at school. This can prove a little clumsy to implement, although it gives the opportunity to amend the regime to cover difficult times of the day.

The advantage of this approach is that the question of medication is addressed in a step-by-step method with parental observations given initial priority so that the family feels in control. The exercise can be abandoned at any point. It provides an opportunity to estimate likely dosing for converting to sustained-release preparations and it is easy to repeat the exercise using immediate-release dexamfetamine, starting with 2.5mg and increasing in 2.5mg steps to test if the child responds preferentially to that.

Alternatively it can, of course, be carried out in a similar way at home using a single dose of a sustained-release preparation, choosing one that has a good range of capsule sizes to allow sensitive determination of milligram dose (5, 10, 15, 20, 25,… or 18, 27, 36,…) with the advantage that this will predict a useful dose for continued use. There is a chance that a long-lasting sustained-release stimulant might produce onset insomnia or an uncomfortable adverse effect such as headache, abdominal pain or overexcitement that then persists for longer than with immediate-release, and puts the family off, but this is very rare. On the other hand, adverse mood change in the afternoon as the dose wears off is less likely. Using sustained-release preparations from the start does have the significant advantage that no medication ever needs to be dispensed in school, avoiding stigmatisation.

The only preparation with which to test for preferential response to sustained-release dexamfetamine that is currently available in the UK is lisdexamfetamine. This, like longer-lasting sustained-release methylphenidate preparations, might cause insomnia in treatment-naïve children (especially young children) and occasionally prejudice willingness to continue. Box 7.5 illustrates an approach to initiating amfetamine medication.

Box 7.5: Initiating dexamfetamine

If this is to follow an unsatisfactory response to methylphenidate it can be substituted the next day; no need to cross taper.

1. Immediate–release dexamfetamine (5mg tablets)

- 2.5mg as initial single dose trial and titrate up according to effect and tolerance (as per methylphenidate), then initiate twice daily regime using optimal dose discovered on single dose trial or change to lisdexamfetamine 30mg daily (see below).

or

- Start 2.5mg twice daily (morning and midday) regime and titrate up by 2.5mg or 5mg intervals per dose with usual maximum daily dose 20mg (some will need up to 40mg).

2. Lisdexamfetamine

- Always start with 30mg daily and titrate accordingly up to 70mg daily. 30mg dose can be lowered by using 20mg capsule.
- Can also adjust dose down by dissolving e.g. a 50mg capsule in a known volume of water (e.g. 50ml) and then halving that volume of solution to yield a 25mg dose providing enormous flexibility of dosing.
- Warn not to bite or crunch capsule. Can be dissolved as above if child cannot swallow.

3. Inform family about side effects

For example decreased appetite, insomnia, GI effects, BP and pulse rate changes etc. (see Chapter 6). Medication can be stopped immediately if appropriate.

Either single-dose trial approach, whether using immediate-release or a sustained-release preparation, requires the ability to communicate easily by phone, text or e-mail with the family after a weekend trial so that advice about the next step can be given.

Progressive titration over days and weeks in both home and school
A widely used alternative is simply to start with a regular, 7-days-a-week, low dose (5mg), two or three times daily, using immediate-release tablets or the lowest available dose of a sustained-release preparation and adjust the dose upwards at intervals of a week or so over a few weeks. This carries a small risk of starting with an unsuitably high dose or starting very low with a long wait until evidence from both home and school for effectiveness is evident. It is important to include weekends or start during school holidays so the parents can see for themselves the effect during the time their child would otherwise be in school.

In practice, this is what many services offer and it works well for the majority of families.

Whichever regime is used to commence treatment, the clinical team of specialist nurses and doctors must provide accessible, prompt and regular follow-up. This will include a combination of face-to-face visits with measurement of effectiveness, direct enquiry to child and parent as to adverse effects, measuring weight, height, blood pressure and pulse, and offering telephone reviews. The aim is to optimise treatment, ensuring a combination of maximal benefit, covering all the difficult times of day while minimising negative effects.

Atomoxetine

An initial trial of atomoxetine is more protracted and its delayed onset of action makes single-dose trials irrelevant. It pays to introduce atomoxetine gradually to minimise side effects (Box 7.6).

The manufacturer's recommended regime is to start at around 0.5mg/kg/day for 1 week and then if this is well tolerated to increase to about 1.2mg/kg/day. An alternative, gentler, but slower approach that minimises adverse effects is to move the daily dose up the capsule sizes on a weekly basis: 10mg daily for a week, followed by 18mg daily, 25mg, 40mg and so forth up to the threshold for effect of 1.2mg/kg/day. The adoption of weekly increases takes advantage of the seven-capsule starter packs. Even with a gentle approach it is necessary to warn about the possibility of short-lived nausea and the small possibility of emergent drowsiness, irritability or abdominal discomfort. With that in mind I usually recommend giving it in the evening, warning that this is different from the morning dose the patient information leaflet in the medicine pack recommends.

Box 7.6: Initiating atomoxetine: two strategies

1. Two-week initiating period

✓ 0.5mg/kg/day for 7 days

✓ then 1.2mg/kg/day

Can increase further to 1.8mg/kg/day if well tolerated and response not yet optimised. Remember child may be slow metaboliser (may not need 1.2mg/kg) or rapid metaboliser (may need twice daily dosing).

Morning dose conventional but evening dose may be more acceptable if nausea or abdominal discomfort.

2. Gradual introduction by capsule size with 7 days at each level

✓ Start with 10mg/day for 7 days

✓ Then 18mg/day, 24mg/day, 40mg/day etc. according to increasing capsule size for 7 days at each dose until 1.2mg/kg/day reached.

Same principle can be followed using liquid.

Reduces likelihood of adverse effects but takes longer.

Either approach can take 3 months to achieve maximum therapeutic effect.

Warn of possible side effects e.g. nausea, GI symptoms, decreased appetite and pulse and BP changes. See Chapter 6 for full side effect profile.

Notes: GI, gastrointestinal; BP, blood pressure.

There will be evidence of effect after 2 weeks at full dose, but the maximal effect can take 12 weeks or more to achieve, which means that a complete trial can ultimately be quite a protracted business. If the 1.2mg/kg/day dose is well tolerated but improvement is felt to be suboptimal, the dose should be increased again to around 1.8mg/kg/day as this may provide additional benefit. Some children who are fast metabolisers also achieve better control on a twice-daily dosage.

Alpha 2 agonists

If these are to be used as monotherapy in individuals for whom stimulants are unsuitable or produce a less than optimal effect then their initiation is a straightforward upward titration at weekly intervals over several weeks.

Clonidine needs to be started with 25µg three times a day, possibly with an additional dose at bedtime if onset insomnia is a pre-existing problem. Titration upwards is then with 25µg intervals per dose. The maximum recommended dose is 0.2mg/day orally for children weighing 27–40.5kg, 0.3mg/day for those weighing 40.5–45kg and 0.4mg/day for those over 45kg. When discontinuing therapy, it should be tapered gradually over 1–2 weeks. The branded preparation and generic alternatives can produce different results, so consistency of preparation is important.

For prolonged-release guanfacine (GXR; Box 7.7), the starting dose is 1mg daily. Drowsiness is a common initial side effect, affecting a third to just under a half of children, but it usually wears off within 3 weeks. Drowsiness permitting, the dose is increased at approximately weekly intervals by 1mg daily towards a target of 0.08–0.12mg/kg/day. This approximates to a maximum dose of 4mg/day for children and up to 7mg/day for teenagers. Recurring drowsiness at each dose increase may occur, so parents and teachers should be informed of this in advance. Children and carers should also be advised that dizziness due to decreased blood pressure may occur, especially on standing up quickly. Maintaining hydration, particularly in hot weather or during exercise, can help. Follow-up in the first year of treatment should be at least every 3 months.

If it is concluded that a trial of an α_2 agonist is unsuccessful, it is recommended that medication should be titrated down 1mg every 3 to 7 days. This is due to the potential risk of a rebound increase in blood pressure. Clinical experience suggests this would be extremely unlikely in children and young people, but it should be advised.

Box 7.7: Initiating prolonged release guanfacine (GXR)

1. Initiating treatment

✓ Once daily, can be morning or evening

✓ 1mg, 2mg, 3mg, 4mg tablets

✓ Begin with 1mg/day and increase by 1mg/day steps to 0.8-1.2mg/kg/day, titrating by effect and tolerance.

✓ That is often 3-4mg/day for children. Teenagers can take up to 7mg/day.

✓ Tablets must be swallowed whole

2. Inform about side effects

✓ Main problem is drowsiness, which affects up to nearly half of all children. Usually wears off after 3 weeks but can recur at each increase in dose so slows rate of initiation.

✓ Some children experience postural hypotension, which again slows titration.

See Chapter 6 for full side effect profile.

3. Stopping medication

Discontinue by tapering off by 1mg every 3-7 days

Measuring progress towards the target

The rule for all ADHD medications is titration – adjusting the dose to obtain a balanced result of effect on symptoms, effect on impairment, tolerance, quality of life and convenience. This is styled an *optimal* dose, derived from the research term 'optimal treatment success' (Setyawan et al. 2015).

Assuming that a target has been set, it will be important to know to what extent this is being achieved, in other words a way of measuring progress is required. For the sake of adherence, this should allow the clinician and family to see 'How far have we got?' rather than 'We're not there yet', which follows if just a target is set with no intermediate steps.

If the chosen approach has been the reduction of all ADHD symptoms, then it is logical to use one of the questionnaires based on the DSM-5 (American Psychiatric Association 2013) items, for example ADHD-RS or SNAP-IV (18-item), which can yield a simple score. Extended versions that include features of oppositional behaviour including the CADDRA ADHD Checklist and the Vanderbilt are another option. The Conners 3 is a rich instrument that taps more than core symptoms, assesses against population norms and is popular in the UK. The longer 26- and 90-item versions of SNAP-IV, which include aspects of common coexisting conditions, are also a possibility.

My preference is to draw up my own version of the ADHD-RS/SNAP-IV (18-item) that takes the DSM-5 items and rewrites them slightly, omitting 'often', specifying tasks as activities set by other people, italicising words requiring specific emphasis such as *seems* (not to listen when spoken to directly) and anglicising the occasional phrase (e.g. has difficulty waiting in a queue).

This can then be scored 0, 1, 2, 3 for each item so a single score (0–54) or two subscale scores for inattention and hyperactivity/impulsivity (each 0–27) can be obtained. Provided that the same rater is asked to complete this scale (parents differ, with mothers usually giving higher scores), a single score gives an idea of progress.

The alternative to this approach is to construct a simple scale for an identified target problem and identify intermediate steps in discussion with both parent and child. A five-point scale, which can be depicted as a ladder, is easiest (Box 7.8). The intermediate steps are important in order to document progress in a positive light.

The top, bottom and intermediate steps are labelled in specific, observable (not inferred), behavioural terms using language that the child understands. It should be possible to obtain a numerical score from the scale. Counting the number of intermediate steps achieved is easy.

A variant of this is a linear analogue scale with identified endpoints (Box 7.9). In each case, one end of the scale is where the child's behaviour was at initial assessment and the

Box 7.8: An informal ladder scale to monitor progress to agreed targets

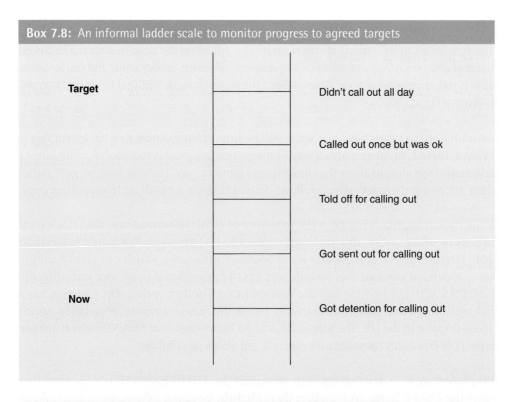

Target

Didn't call out all day

Called out once but was ok

Told off for calling out

Got sent out for calling out

Now

Got detention for calling out

Box 7.9: Examples of a simple linear scale

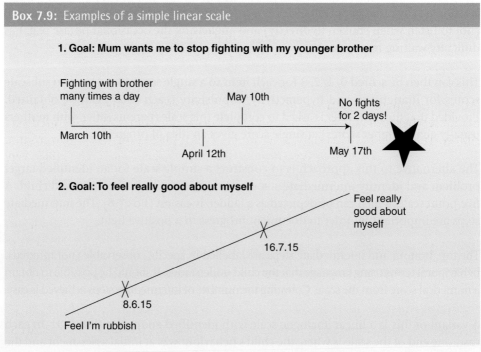

1. Goal: Mum wants me to stop fighting with my younger brother

Fighting with brother many times a day

May 10th

No fights for 2 days!

March 10th

April 12th

May 17th

2. Goal: To feel really good about myself

Feel really good about myself

16.7.15

8.6.15

Feel I'm rubbish

other end is the identified target. A linear scale can be marked with a cross by the child and the distance from baseline measured with a ruler if necessary. Alternatively, progress can be marked by date along a line.

The medicine's effect is described as 'helping the child to achieve'. The questions at appointment should be, for example, 'Is it working well enough?', 'How useful has it been so far in getting to what we want?' Using this approach brings psychological factors derived from behaviour therapy practice into play, such as labelling a target in explicit quantifiable terms, emphasising praise, recognition of incremental achievement and so forth. The pivotal feature, however, is getting a simple numerical value that reflects how treatment is progressing so that the rationale for titrating medication doses can be seen by all.

Obtaining information from a teacher about progress follows the same principle. Variation between subject teachers in secondary schools is a well-known problem and some discussion as to which teacher should be asked is wise. If the main issue is observed classroom behaviour, the DSM-5 item scales, as above, will suffice, but they do not have the same face validity for teachers as the SKAMP, the last ten items of the 90-item version of the SNAP-IV, which can be scored 0, 1, 2, 3 for each item and thus yields a single score (0–30). Similarly the Conners 3 scales appear to be more acceptable to most teachers.

The Conners 3-Teacher (3-T) exists in both long and short versions, and which to choose depends on the willingness of the teacher to fill it in. Both are useful for picking up issues such as peer relationships in addition to core ADHD symptoms. If repeated measures are needed at frequent intervals, the Conners 3 ADHD Index (3AI) is a 10-item scale useful for monitoring major aspects.

If the chosen main focus of treatment in the school setting is a single issue, then asking for teacher feedback on the five-point or linear-scale approach can be used very simply. The target (such as calling out in class, poor integration in the playground, avoiding detention, handing in work) and intermediate steps may be identified very straightforwardly.

If the main issue is underachievement then this can only be assessed at longer intervals once inattention has been corrected, because the best measure is, unsurprisingly, achievement in terms of marks or grades. The same is true for self-organisation and homework completion when these are lead problems. In such instances a qualitative report by the teacher may be more useful than simply pursuing questionnaire scores.

A further consideration is titration across the day. The sustained-release methylphenidate medications differ importantly in their release of active medication (see Appendix 5) and it is important to match this to situational fluctuations in behaviour across the day. Parents should be asked about morning routines, school journeys and homework demands, but they will not always know about issues across the school day and the Dundee Difficult Times of Day scale is useful in that respect. This is an important but often neglected aspect of titration.

Problems often arise when stimulant control cannot be achieved in the early morning or evening. Behavioural difficulties before breakfast cannot usually be resolved by stimulants alone, and substitution or co-prescription of a prolonged-release α_2 agonist (or its use alone) or a switch to atomoxetine may be indicated. Difficulties with weak control from OROS methylphenidate early in the school day or poor control in the late afternoon or evening can be addressed by adding an immediate-release dose of the same stimulant in the morning or mid-afternoon accordingly ('topping and tailing'). Some families report a smoother and longer effect from lisdexamfetamine.

Tailoring both medication and preparation to the individual child is key.

Titration to what point?

Although conventional guidance for stimulants is to continue titrating the dose upwards until an optimal dose is reached, this can mean extending the dose beyond the range approved by regulatory authorities. NICE (2008) and the American Academy of Child and Adolescent Psychiatry Work Group (Pliszka 2007) have recognised this, but some clinicians consider themselves restricted to a 'licensed' dose. They need not, as a 'licence' is a marketing authorisation for a manufacturer, not a prescriber. Hill (2005) addresses guidance on the topic in more detail.

Some clinicians have used very high doses of OROS methylphenidate to produce benefit without adverse cardiovascular effect (up to 270mg/day in Stevens et al. 2010). This study, like others, found no relationship between oral dose and blood level. Although higher doses than those 'licensed' are not uncommonly needed, the possibility of overlooking a preferential dexamfetamine responder needs to be borne in mind. It is also vital in a clinical setting to be clear that the difficulties remaining are due to ADHD and not part of a comorbid problem. Box 7.10 can be a useful aide memoire when faced by reports of ongoing difficulty.

A similar problem arises when prescribing atomoxetine by weight to large teenagers when this predicts a higher daily dose than the recommended 100mg. I suggest that it is appropriate to proceed cautiously in order to obtain a daily dose of 1.2mg/kg/day, the threshold for efficacy. Splitting a large dose between morning and evening dosing may be helpful.

Box 7.10: It isn't working well enough

Before increasing dose or changing medication, ask yourself

What does this mean?

✓ What exactly isn't working – are expectations appropriate?

✓ Does everyone, including school, agree it isn't working? Is there enough information to know for sure?

✓ Is it working well at any time of the day?

Is this an adherence issue?

✓ Is the medication being given regularly?

✓ Is it being taken (and swallowed)?

✓ Is the process being undermined by adverse comments from other family members, peers, teachers?

Am I on the right track?

✓ Is the diagnosis right?

✓ Am I missing comorbidity (anxiety causing restlessness, ASD producing inattentiveness etc.)?

✓ Is this another way of saying that side effects make it too unpleasant to continue?

✓ Is there something going on in the life of the patient and family?

Before switching medication

✓ Have I titrated properly?

✓ Is this the optimal preparation for delivering medication across the day?

✓ Is this the maximum dose?

Managing side effects

Parents appreciate being told in advance about common adverse effects (Gajria et al. 2014), but it makes sense to do so in conjunction with a statement about the positive main effects. Parents report being motivated by hearing about these. It is worth making the point that medicines can be stopped promptly (or at any rate swiftly in the case of the α_2 agonists) if unacceptable adverse effects emerge.

A balanced analysis of the risks of adverse effects is provided by the European Guidelines Group (Graham et al. 2011) and findings since then have supported their conclusions. Unwanted effects of medication are the commonest reason for poor adherence to medication (Gajria et al. 2014) and their management is thus crucial for an optimal treatment outcome.

It is more fruitful to ask directly about subjective side effects than wait for them to be raised spontaneously (Lee et al. 2013). A valuable approach is to ask older children to complete a questionnaire asking about both positive and negative effects of medication. A clinic can devise their own, modelled perhaps on the approach described by Cox et al. (2015).

Slowed weight gain secondary to appetite suppression by stimulants can often be countered by altering the timing of medication and allowing extra food in the evening or at breakfast.

Sleep problems associated with stimulants may be eased by using a sustained-release preparation with shorter release time, but on occasion, onset insomnia seems simply to be associated with stimulant prescription itself. Sometimes children will use a tablet, phone or laptop to while away the time before sleep and this can be counterproductive as the light emission inhibits endogenous melatonin release. Exogenous melatonin, usually 2–10mg 1 hour before desired sleep onset time is a widely used method of inducing sleep onset (with digital tablet or phone use either prohibited or used with a blue-light filter app during this time). If it proves insufficient, many families will try an over-the-counter remedy such as a sedative antihistamine although this approach carries the risk of drowsiness the next morning (until the stimulant counteracts this). Traditionally, immediate-release clonidine 50–200µg 1 hour before bed is widely used. Trazodone 50mg is an alternative approach, should clonidine be insufficient and, although it is said to be associated with a risk of priapism (which one might think a risk given that this is also a rare side effect of stimulants), I have never seen this occur.

A side effect that can be problematic for teenagers is the subjective sense that they have lost their social spontaneity. This seems to be more than no longer being the class clown or otherwise entertaining others by impulsive behaviour and is not obviously a consequence of excessive dosing. For those on methylphenidate, it appears that some will recover their sense of spontaneity and social engagement without losing treatment benefit if switched to lisdexamfetamine.

It is hard to know what to do for abdominal pain associated with stimulants. Sometime switching preparation or stimulant or changing to atomoxetine helps, but there is no guarantee.

Tics are not as likely to be caused by medication as is generally assumed (Roessner et al. 2006; Cohen et al. 2015) and existing tics are not usually affected by stimulants. In perhaps 10% of individuals they will worsen, but after 12 weeks most of these will have subsided (Tourette Syndrome Study Group 2002) and continuing exacerbation, although reversible, is confined to 5% or less of children with tics. Ordinarily, atomoxetine is prescribed when tics are present as it is less likely to exacerbate tics, although this is not a complete guarantee (Graham et al. 2011), but prolonged-release guanfacine has the capacity to suppress tics and should be considered when tics and ADHD coexist.

A severe tic disorder or Tourette syndrome with severe comorbid ADHD may require a tic suppressant such as aripiprazole or risperidone as well as stimulant medication.

Cardiovascular issues are addressed in Chapter 9.

Adherence

Failure to take medication as prescribed is rife and under-recognised. Even in the well-supervised children in the Multimodal Treatment of Attention Deficit Hyperactivity disorder (MTA) study, 25% had fewer than half of their saliva samples positive for medication, even though less than 3% were non-adherent by parental report (Pappadopulos et al. 2009). Rates of failure rise with time and, at 3 years after initiation, rather less than half will continue with recommended medication (Atzori 2009). Not surprisingly, the problem is greater with adolescents than children, because parental authority and supervision is less.

Generally speaking, the following have been shown to help:

- education of both parent and patient about their medication
- use of sustained-release preparations
- incorporating dosing into daily household rhythms
- active management of side effects
- a problem-orientated approach
- more frequent follow-up
- secure arrangements for transition to adult services

In the context of a follow-up appointment it pays to address the child directly or interview an adolescent on their own and convey your expectation that they will miss doses by asking what happens when they do, as if simply checking for effect.

Failure to respond

Some issues have already been covered or are obvious:

- wrong diagnosis
- wrong medication in a preferential responder
- inadequate dosing
- not taking the medication as prescribed
- clinician and family working to different goals

The important principle is to avoid blame and generate a joint problem-solving attitude. Box 7.10 helps to review the situation with the family.

A structured approach

Boxes 7.11, 7.12 and 7.13 are reminders of the general principles for using medication in the management of ADHD, how to decide if response is optimised and routine monitoring at every clinic review.

You may also wish to look back at Box 7.3 to review recommended practice around choice of medications and when to change from one to another.

Choosing between non-stimulants

There is little science to inform choice between atomoxetine and prolonged-release guanfacine. In theory, if a child has not shown a response to dexamfetamine, atomoxetine should be unlikely to succeed because both block the effect on the noradrenaline reuptake transporter. Prolonged-release guanfacine (GXR) would be preferred in the presence of tics because it can suppress these. In my experience, GXR is nearly always neutral as far as appetite and weight are concerned (even though the Summary of Product Characteristics (SPC) mentions weight gain as an adverse effect). When considering ADHD associated with autism spectrum disorder (ASD) or learning disability, remember that atomoxetine is available in liquid form.

Box 7.11: General principles of using stimulant medication in ADHD

✓ Know the pharmacokinetic profile of blood levels across the day and the mechanism of release from different sustained-release stimulant preparations. Match release profile to needs of child (see Appendix 5).

✓ Titrate dose gradually upwards until goal attained or no further clinical improvement, provided child is not over-medicated and side effects are tolerable. There are no standard doses of stimulants.

✓ Titrate more slowly when ASD, tic disorder, epilepsy, anxiety or eating disorder are comorbid conditions.

✓ Actively enquire about, monitor and document side effects and ameliorate or reduce dose if not possible.

✓ Follow progress regularly and contact family promptly after any dose change.

✓ Manage ongoing prescription within a shared care protocol with GP. When GP declines shared care they should nevertheless be informed about current medication.

Source: Adapted from NICE (2008).

Box 7.12: How do I decide if the response is good enough?

Measurement of change from baseline is the key: 'is he better?' is not enough. Ask family, child/young person and school/college.

Either

Evaluate according to agreed target using simple five-point or linear scale or key problem resolution (e.g. not suspended from school) as well as general clinical impression.

or

Measure core symptoms using e.g. ADHD rating scale or SNAP:

✓ A total score of 27 or less (a mean item score of <1.5) is conventionally taken as a clinically significant response.

✓ A total score of 18 or less (an average item score of <1.0) implies normalisation unless there are major outliers.

Ask about negative effects directly.

Ensure child is not over-medicated.

Ask about different times of day and different settings.

Box 7.13: Actions at every follow-up clinic

Consider obtaining reports or ratings from school and parent well beforehand (not in the waiting room).

Talk to child as well as parent.

Assess progress

✓ Ask directly about positive effects and contrast with days when medication omitted.

✓ Ask directly about side effects and take steps to ameliorate.

✓ Ask about negative aspects: teasing by siblings, conflict over taking medicine.

✓ Check height and weight, plot on growth chart.

✓ Check pulse and blood pressure and compare with normal values (Appendices 2 and 3).

✓ Review impairment secondary to known or emerging comorbid difficulties and treat if necessary.

✓ Provide one piece of information about ADHD or medication.

Switching medication

Moving from one stimulant to the other is easy and can be done on consecutive days. Note that a given dose of either dexamfetamine or methylphenidate does not accurately predict what the corresponding dose of the alternative will be.

Switching from stimulant to atomoxetine or GXR can be done by rapidly cross-tapering over 2 weeks (Cardo et al. 2013) or by simply maintaining the dose of stimulant while increasing the dose of the non-stimulant incrementally. There seems to be little to choose between the two approaches.

Combining medications

Poor response to one medication usually indicates a need to switch rather than combine, but combining stimulants with atomoxetine or α_2 adrenergic agonists is increasingly used, albeit off-label, to enable symptom control in the evenings and early mornings when a non-stimulant is insufficient on its own. The use of clonidine at night in order to facilitate sleep onset has a long history and is straightforward.

Such combinations appear safe (previous concerns about combining stimulants with clonidine have subsided), but common sense suggests it is wise to monitor cardiovascular effects in particular.

Supplementing a main medicine with an immediate-release preparation to cover difficult points in the day is common practice. It makes sense to use an immediate-release form of the same medication shown to provide optimal response (i.e. dexamfetamine to supplement lisdexamfetamine).

Comorbidity

The effect of comorbid conditions on choice or use of medications is discussed in Chapter 11.

One further issue is the difficulty in balancing stimulant or atomoxetine treatment for ADHD against the possibility of misuse to restrict appetite when treating ADHD comorbid with anorexia nervosa. It can be done, but requires extremely careful monitoring of adherence and also potassium levels in those who induce vomiting. A mutually trusting open relationship between clinician, patient and family is crucial. Alpha-2 adrenergic agonists may have a part to play, although reading information online that guanfacine can cause weight gain may lead to a reluctance on the part of the patient to consider it. In real life, marked weight gain seems very rare and may simply occur because a patient was previously on stimulants that have been stopped.

Preschool children

Guidelines advocate caution when medication is used in the under 6 years age group and nearly all ADHD medications are off-label in this group. Dexamfetamine is authorised in the UK for children of 3 years and over. NICE guidelines (NICE 2008) state that 'drug treatment is not recommended for preschool children', and the advocated treatment of choice is parent management support.However, the American Academy of Pediatrics Clinical Practice Guideline (2011) sanctions the use of methylphenidate in this age group if behavioural measures fail. This derives from the Preschool ADHD Treatment Study (PATS) study (Greenhill et al. 2006), which showed that methylphenidate can be helpful, albeit with less efficacy than with older children and with a higher rate of adverse effects. Similarly, atomoxetine will work in 5-year-olds, although rather less effectively than in older children (Kratochvil et al. 2011).

Given that hyperactivity is a more prominent problem in preschool children, a number of clinicians have favoured a trial of clonidine rather than stimulants in the very young, and the availability of prolonged-release guanfacine may now prove useful.

Swallowing solid medication has historically been an issue in young school-age children and some of those with autism, intellectual disability or physical swallowing diffiuclties, but liquid preparations of both immediate-release methylphenidate and dexamfetamine have recently become available. Atomoxetine oral solution is available, and lisdexamfetamine can be dissolved in water. The bead preparations of sustained-release methylphenidate can be sprinkled on apple sauce or equivalent. In the USA, the patch for methylphenidate and liquid sustained-release methyphenidate are options.

Continuing medication

Although the benefits of medication on behaviour and some aspects of neuropsychological competence can be seen quickly, longer-term use brings wider gains, particularly for the use of medication combined with non-pharmacological interventions, on academic achievement, social functioning and quality of life and self-esteem (Arnold et al. 2015; Harpin et al. 2016). Longer duration of medication is associated with greater academic achievement (Scheffler et al. 2009).

Medication during childhood does not increase the subsequent rate of substance misuse in young adulthood (Wilens et al. 2011; Molina et al. 2013).

It is often believed that continuing active treatment of ADHD lessens the chance of social misbehaviour, especially when this is impulsive. Evidence to justify this is hard to find, but a Swedish study (Lichtenstein et al. 2012) showed offending by older adolescents and adults to be reduced when on medication for ADHD.

Stopping medication

Termination of medication by the clinician will be because it is not tolerated or is no longer needed or to test whether it is still needed. A clue as to whether a stimulant is still useful is to ask the patient, presuming that some medication days will be missed, 'What happens when you miss a dose…', or asking about times when medication cover is absent (evenings or weekends for those on school-day-only treatment). Many families run out of medication, which also provides an opportunity to observe withdrawal.

The situation with non-stimulants is less clear cut and it makes sense to have a planned withdrawal every year or so to test continuing effect using information from patient, parents and school.

Development of autonomy

The exceptionally high rate of medication discontinuation in late adolescence (Wong et al. 2009) is shocking given that the spontaneous rate of improvement in the condition over the same period is only slow. Although some of this is because of inadequate transition arrangements, much of the reason is because young people take the matter of medication into their own hands, growing beyond parental control, leaving school and making judgements about their own mental health needs, often with less than ideal information. The contract with the clinician changes as autonomy passes to the young adult and the primacy of their subjective concerns. Furthermore, first encounters with an adult psychiatric clinic can be alarming, especially for those who have been looked after by paediatric services.

To counteract this, a progressive approach to increasing adolescents' understanding of and responsibility for medication can be initiated from the early teens. Addressing them directly during follow-up appointments and asking them to complete questionnaires about ADHD symptoms and medication effects to elicit any unvoiced concerns is sensible. Giving them some say in dosing schedules or preparations in the light of their subjective account as well as feedback from teachers and parents is can be done gradually over time from about age 14 years. Explaining to parents that their offspring will make their own decisions in any case at 16–18 years can defuse the concern that they will exploit the situation. See Chapter 13 for more discussion of how to support young people.

Conclusion

The use of medication in the treatment of ADHD is an art, informed by science. It is a collaborative exercise involving clinician, parents, teachers and, most importantly, the child or young person patient. There is no standard medicine or dose, but a continuing process of adjustments to treatment in light of individual progress reported by multiple sources of information. This change should be measured and its extent appreciated by all. The approach must always be aiming for the best possible and not just 'good enough'.

Summary

- Parents and children are often anxious about using medication for ADHD. Be prepared to discuss medication at some length.

- Provide written information about medicines. Explain the main effects before side effects. Refer to standard guidelines or quality websites.

- Dependency on stimulants prescribed for childhood ADHD is exceptionally rare (if it ever occurs), and the prescription of stimulants may even reduce later substance misuse.

- Use formal or informal scales that can be understood by all family members. Share scores or ratings on these with them. This will improve adherence.

- Unless contraindicated, use stimulants first.

- Initiate on a step-by-step basis with a single dose trial or very early follow-up of low-dose extended release.

- Setting goals and targets enables everyone to understand and measure how much progress towards these is being made.

- Do not be satisfied simply with some general improvement.

- Titrate dose progressively, testing against target and adverse effects.

- Early and regular follow-up is very important.

- Consider the effect across the day and choose methylphenidate preparations accordingly.

- Switch to another stimulant rather than serially substitute alternative preparations.

- Introduce non-stimulants gradually.

- Prolong initial treatment with atomoxetine for maximal benefit.

- Consider guanfacine if there are coexisting major tics.

- Manage side effects actively.

- Consider whether rigid adherence to marketing authorisations ('licences') is in the interests of the child.

- Consider various reasons for failure to achieve target. Poor adherence is very common.

- Help adolescents develop towards autonomy in the management of their medication.

Resources: Assessment Scales

The basic 18-item, extended 26-item and full 90-item versions of SNAP-IV are available free from the ADHD toolkit on www.shared-care.ca. The SNAP-IV (26 items), ADHD-RS and SKAMP scales can be obtained free from CADDRA in their ADHD Assessment Toolkit (www.caddra.ca).

The full ADHD-RS scales and scoring manual (DuPaul et al. 2016) can be purchased from Guilford Press (www.guilford.com), but a number of virtually identical symptom lists are freely available online from CADDRA, for example.

The Conners 3 parent, teacher and self-completion scales can be purchased from Pearson Education (www.pearsonclinical.co.uk).

The first (and very adequate) edition of the 2002 NICHQ Vanderbilt Assessment Scales can be downloaded free from www.nichq.org. The second 2011 edition can be purchased from the American Academy of Pediatrics (www.shop.aap.org).

The Dundee-Difficult Times Of Day Scale (D-DTODS) is available free from www.healthcareimprovementscotland.org.

References

American Psychiatric Association (2013) *Diagnostic and statistical manual of mental disorders,* 5th edn. Arlington, VA: American Psychiatric Association Publishers.

American Academy of Pediatrics (2011) ADHD clinical practice guideline for the diagnosis, evaluation and treatment of attention-deficit/hyperactivity disorder in children and adolescents. *Pediatrics* 128: 1007–1022, doi:10.1542/peds.2011-2654.

Arnold LE, Hodgkins P, Caci H et al. (2015) Effect of treatment modality on long-term outcomes in attention-deficit/hyperactivity disorder: A systematic review *PLoS One* 10(2): e0116407, doi:10.1371/journal.pone.0116407.

Atzori P, Usala T, Carucci S et al. (2009) Predictive factors for persistent use and compliance of immediate-release methylphenidate: A 36-month naturalistic study. *J Child Adolesc Psychopharmacol* 19: 673–681, doi:10.1089/cap.2008.0146.

Cardo E, Porsdal V, Quail D et al. (2013) Fast vs. slow switching from stimulants to atomoxetine in children and adolescents with attention-deficit/hyperactivity disorder. *J Child Adolesc Psychopharmacol* 23: 252–261, doi:10.1089/cap.2012.0027.

Cohen S, Mulqueen J, Ferracioli-Oda E et al. (2015) Meta-analysis: Risk of tics associated with psychostimulant use in randomized, placebo-controlled trials. *J Am Acad Child Adolesc Psychiatry* 54: 728–736, doi:10.1016/j.jaac.2015.06.011.

Cox DJ, Davis MT, Cox BS et al. (2015) Quantifying the relationship between perceived consequences of ADHD medication and its usage. *J Attent Disord* 19: 78–83, doi:10.1177/1087054712452913.

Danckaerts M, Sonuga-Barke E, Banaschewski T et al. (2010) The quality of life of children with attention-deficit/hyperactivity disorder: A systematic review. *Eur Child Adolesc Psychiatry* 19: 83–105, doi:10.007/s00787-009-0046-3.

DuPaul GJ, Power TJ, Anastopoulos AD, Reid R (2016) *ADHD rating scale–5 for children and adolescents.* New York, NY: Guilford Press.

Gajria K, Lu M, Sikirica V et al. (2014) Adherence, persistence, and medication discontinuation in patients with attention-deficit/hyperactivity disorder – a systematic literature review. *Neuropsychiat Dis Treatment* 10: 1543–1569, doi:10.2147/NDT.S65721.

Graham J, Banaschewski T, Buitelaar J et al. (2011) European guidelines on managing adverse effects of medication for ADHD. *Eur Child Adolesc Psychiatry* 20: 17–37, doi:10.1007/s00787-010-0140-6.

Greenhill L, Kollins S, Abikoff H et al. (2006) Efficacy and safety of immediate release methylphenidate treatment for preschoolers with ADHD. *J Am Acad Child Adolesc Psychiatry* 45: 1284–1293, doi:10.1097/01.chi.0000235077.32661.61.

Harpin V, Mazzone L, Raynaud J-P et al. (2016) Long-term outcomes of ADHD: A systematic review of self-esteem and social functioning. *J Attent Disord* 20: 295–305, doi:10.1177/1087054713486516.

Hill P (2005) Off-licence and off-label prescribing in children: Litigation fears for physicians. *Arch Dis Child* 90(Suppl 1): i17–18, doi:10.1136/adc.2004.058867.

Kratochvil CJ, Vaughan BS, Stoner JA et al. (2011) A double-blind placebo-controlled study of atomoxetine in young children with ADHD. *Pediatrics* 127: e862–e868, doi:10.1542/peds.2010-0825.

Lee M-S, Lee SI, Hong SD et al. (2013) Two different solicitation methods for obtaining information on adverse events associated with methylphenidate in adolescents: A 12-week multicenter, open-label, study. *J Child Adolesc Psychopharmacol* 23: 22–27, doi:10.1089/cap.2012.0018.

Lichtenstein P, Halldner L, Zetterqvist J et al. (2012) Medication for attention-deficit-hyperactivity disorder and criminality. *N Eng J Med* 367: 2006–2014, doi:10.1056/NEJMoa1203241.

Molina BSG, Hinshaw SP, Arnold LE (2013) Adolescent substance use in the Multimodal Treatment Study of Attention-Deficit/Hyperactivity Disorder (ADHD) (MTA) as a function of childhood ADHD, random assignment to childhood treatments, and subsequent medication. *J Am Acad Child Adolesc Psychiatry* 52: 250–263, doi:10.1016/j.jaac2012.12.014.

NICE (2008) *Attention deficit hyperactivity disorder: Diagnosis and management. NICE Clinical Guidelines* [CG72], https://www.nice.org.uk/guidance/cg72.

Pappadopulos E, Jensen PS, Chait AR et al. (2009) Medication adherence in the MTA: Saliva methylphenidate samples versus parent report and mediating effect of concomitant behavioral treatment. *J Am Acad Child Adolesc Psychiatry* 48: 501–510, doi:10.1097/CHI.0b013e31819c23ed.

Pelham W, Hoza B, Kipp HL et al. (1997) Effects of methylphenidate and expectancy of ADHD children's performance, self-evaluations, persistence, and attributions on a cognitive task. *Exp Clin Psychopharmacol* 5: 3–13, doi:10.1037/1064-1297.5.1.3.

Pliszka S and the AACAP Work Group on Quality Issues (2007) Practice parameter for the assessment and treatment of children and adolescents with attention-deficit/hyperactivity disorder. *J Am Acad Child Adolesc Psychiatry* 46: 894–921, doi:10.1097/chi.0b013e318054e724.

Roessner V, Robatzek M, Knapp G et al. (2006) First-onset tics in patients with attention deficit hyperactivity disorder: Impact of stimulants. *Dev Med Child Neurol* 48: 616–621, doi:10.1017/S0012162206001290.

Scheffler RM, Brown TT, Fulton BD et al. (2009) Positive association between attention-deficit/hyperactivity disorder medication use and academic achievement during elementary school. *Pediatrics* 123: 1273–1279, doi:10.1542/peds.2008-1597.

Setyawan J, Fridman M, Hodgkins P et al. (2015) Relationship between symptom impairment and treatment outcome in children and adolescents with attention-deficit hyperactivity disorder: A physician perspective. *ADHD Attent Defic Hyperact Disord* 7: 75–87, doi:10.1007/s12402-014-0143-0.

Stevens JR, George RA, Fusillo S et al. (2010) Plasma methylphenidate concentrations in youths treated with high-dose osmotic release oral system formulation. *J Child Adolesc Psychopharmacol* 20: 49–54, doi:10.1089/cap.2008.0128.

Tourette's Syndrome Study Group (2002) Treatment of ADHD in children with tics. *Neurology* 58: 527–536, doi:10.1212/WNL.58.4.527.

Volkow N, Swanson J (2008) Does childhood treatment of ADHD with stimulant medication affect substance abuse in adulthood? *Am J Psychiatry* 165: 553–555, doi:10.1176/app.ajp.2008.08020237.

Weiss MD, Wasdell MB, Bomben MM et al. (2006) Sleep hygiene and melatonin treatment for children and adolescents with ADHD andinitial insomnia. *J Am Acad Child Adolesc Psychiatry* 45: 512–519, doi:10.1097/01 chi.0000205706.78818.ef.

Wilens TE, Martelon M, Joshi G et al. (2011) Does ADHD predict substance-use disorders? A 10-year follow-up study of young adults with ADHD. *J Am Acad Child Adolesc Psychiatry* 50: 543–553, doi:10.1016/j.jaac.2011.01.021.

Wong IC, Asherson P, Bilbow A et al. 2009 Cessation of attention deficit hyperactivity disorder drugs in the young (CADDY) – a pharmacoepidemiological and qualitative study. *Health Technol Assess* 13(50): 1–120, doi:10.3310/hta13500.

Zulauf CA, Sprich SE, Safren SA, Wilens TE (2014) The complicated relationship between attention-deficit/hyperactivity disorder and substance use disorders. *Curr Psychiatry Rep* 16: 436, doi:10.1007/s11920-013-0436-6.

Chapter 8

Monitoring growth

Val Harpin

Monitoring growth is important in all children. Clearly, the aim is for all children to reach their optimal final height and weight in adulthood. However, there are also other relevant issues. A child who is underweight may be malnourished, resulting in anaemia and immune deficiency. An overweight child is at risk from raised blood pressure, type 2 diabetes, psychological problems and, in adult life, from heart disease and stroke.

Children with ADHD come in all shapes and sizes, varying from underweight to over-weight for their age, and we need to take this into account when monitoring the effect of the medications we may use on their growth.

What is known about the effect of ADHD medications on growth?

More than 40 years ago, Safer et al. (1972) reported that long-term stimulant treatment of children decreased growth velocity and, as the use of stimulant medications increased in the next 2 decades, further studies investigated the extent, persistence and possible mechanisms of stimulant-induced growth suppression. It was observed that the effect on weight was usually seen in the first few months of treatment and then often settled. The effect on height, however, was often not apparent until later. From these studies, the loss of expected growth in height was estimated to be around 1cm per year for children treated continuously for at least 3 years with daily doses above 20mg of methylphenidate. By contrast, Klein and Mannuzza (1988) found no difference in final height between young adults who had taken an average daily dose of 45mg of methylphenidate for 5–6 years and untreated controls.

However, at this time, methylphenidate treatment was often stopped before puberty, and most of these young people had stopped treatment before 13 years of age. The Multimodal Treatment (MTA) trial of children with attention deficit disorder also followed growth during treatment and confirmed that growth could be affected (MTA Cooperative Group 2004; Swanson et al. 2007).

For a more detailed review of the literature on the effects of stimulant medication and atomoxetine on growth see Poulton (2005) and Vitiello (2008). In conclusion, continuous use of stimulant medication appears to result, on average, in a loss of height of approximately 1cm per year in the first 1–3 years of treatment. Again, loss in weight was reported to be maximal in the early months of treatment and then less dramatic. Atomoxetine also caused reduction in weight and height, but possibly to a lesser degree. The effects were dose-dependent. The major cause of the growth effects is felt to be decreased appetite, resulting in decreased intake, but other mechanisms cannot be ruled out.

Although these findings overall were not felt to prohibit medication use, recommendations were made that growth should be monitored during treatment with stimulant and non-stimulant medications.

Clinical experience suggests that, although many children and young people are able to take stimulant medication and atomoxetine without significant long-term effects on their growth, there are a minority who appear to be more sensitive to the medication-induced growth suppression and need more careful monitoring and support.

Monitoring growth

First, every clinician should have access to an accurate weighing scale, and children should be weighed in light clothing and without shoes. Measuring height needs training and, again, accurate equipment. When measuring a child's height, the child must be standing symmetrically with their back against the wall, heels together, and head erect in a neutral position. The marker is then gently lowered to touch the head.

Having taken a good measurement, care needs to be taken to plot it accurately on a chart. It is amazing how often measurements are plotted incorrectly. Using a chart ensures that expected growth is taken into account rather than just the last measurement. Electronic growth charts are now becoming increasingly available. (http://www.healthforallchildren. com/growth-online), which will increase accuracy.

Weight and height should be recorded at baseline and at every following visit before starting any medication to establish a growth trajectory before adding medication into the equation. Plotting the height and weight at every visit allows the clinician to compare future changes in weight and height with what would be expected for that child.

If the initial growth trajectory is not within the expected range this should be investigated first. A diary of dietary intake including both type of food and approximate amounts is needed. Physical examination may reveal an unsuspected cause of poor growth and, rarely, blood investigations may be needed. Referral to a paediatrician and/or dietician may be helpful if your own team does not include paediatric expertise.

It is also important to recognise if the child/young person was overweight before starting medication. Sometimes, families have resorted to frequent snacks to calm and occupy an overactive child. In those who are overweight, management of ADHD sometimes results in eating fewer snacks and eating healthier meals and can result in the child reaching a normal body mass index. Weight loss or lack of weight gain may then be a positive outcome.

In those who start off underweight or are on a low height centile, particular care is needed to ensure that the child is not becoming nutritionally compromised and to protect final height.

Starting medication

Whenever a medication that may reduce appetite and compromise growth is started, parents should be made aware of this, and of course other potential side effects. Advice about good nutrition with healthy but high-calorie meals should be given as part of starting medication. You may find it helpful to work with your local dietician to develop a leaflet to give to families at this point.

NICE guidelines (NICE 2008) make recommendations for the monitoring of growth for children and young people taking the ADHD medications methylphenidate, atomoxetine, dexamfetamine or lysdexamfetamine:

- Height should be measured every 6 months, while weight should be measured 3 and 6 months after drug treatment has started and every 6 months thereafter.

- Height and weight in children and young people should be plotted on a growth chart and reviewed by the healthcare professional responsible for their treatment.

If there is concern about weight loss, more frequent monitoring is needed and strategies to help should be implemented. Always ask if the child/young person is experiencing loss of appetite and if they are feeling nauseous after medication, which will further limit food intake.

Strategies to reduce weight loss or manage decreased weight gain in children include the following:

- Take medication either with or after food, rather than before meals (this should decrease loss of appetite at the time of meals and nausea).

- Take additional meals/snacks early in the morning or late in the evening when the stimulant effects of the drug have worn off. These should be high in calories but also nutritious snacks, not 'junk'. It is always wise to check with parents what the family usually eat and can access, (i.e. where they can shop and what they can afford).

- Obtain dietary advice. Initially, using a leaflet you have discussed with your local dietician may be enough.

- Consume high-calorie foods of good nutritional value at all meals.

The NICE guidelines (2008) also state: 'If growth is significantly affected by drug treatment (i.e. the child or young person has not met the height expected for their age), the option of a planned break in treatment over school holidays should be considered to allow "catch-up" growth to occur.'

This may not be possible for many families, as holiday times are often extremely stressful. All other options should be tried first, but, sometimes, targeted medication use in the holidays is helpful and welcomed by families.

If medication is very beneficial and growth is poor, referral to a dietician and the use of milk or juice-based food supplement drinks should be considered. In addition, vitamins and iron supplements may be needed if a food diary demonstrates insufficient intake.

Other causes of poor growth

Children and young people with ADHD may also develop other reasons for poor growth, so if growth suppression seems greater than expected and the usual methods to improve growth do not help, referral for a specialist paediatric opinion may be needed.

Food additives and ADHD

It is also helpful to discuss additives and colours in the diet. Many families may have read about them. Additives can increase overactivity in children with and without ADHD (McCann et al. 2007), but they do not of course actually cause ADHD. Nonetheless, removing them from the diet of children with ADHD may help to decrease activity levels to some extent and be helpful alongside other management strategies. It is helpful to give parents a list of additives to exclude. Occasionally, particular foods, including sometimes apparently healthy ones such as fruit, increase overactivity in some children. Again, exclusion from the diet can be helpful. Sonuga-Barke et al. (2013) performed a meta-analysis and found some difference in ADHD symptoms, but they felt this was small and may be limited to those with food sensitivities.

Free fatty acid supplementation

The same review article also considered the use of free fatty acid supplementation for ADHD symptoms. The authors concluded that there was evidence of benefit but that the effect was small when raters were blinded to the treatment. More research looking at wider outcomes and in a placebo-controlled double-blind design may be useful.

Summary

Growth should be monitored in children and young people diagnosed with ADHD both before and during treatment. As appetite and growth suppression is caused by some medications for ADHD, the following measures should be taken:

- Discuss the possibility of reduced appetite and growth suppression before starting the medication.

- Take steps to reduce the likelihood of problems occurring.

- Measure weight and height carefully and regularly, and record them accurately.

- If problems begin, implement further steps to try to improve appetite and growth.

- If problems persist, carefully assess ongoing risks versus the benefits of continuing medication in discussion with the child and family.

- Consider changing or stopping medication.

- Always remember that poor growth can be an indicator of many illnesses in childhood and consider investigating this further.

References

Klein RG, Mannuzza S (1988) Hyperactive boys almost grown up. III. Methylphenidate effects on ultimate height. *Arch Gen Psychiatry* 45: 1131–1134, doi:10.1001/archpsyc.1988.01800360079012.

McCann D, Barrett A, Cooper A et al. (2007) Food additives and hyperactive behaviour in 3-year-old and 8/9-year-old children in the community: a randomised, double-blind, placebo-controlled trial. *Lancet* 3: 1560–1567, doi:10.1016/S0140-6736(07)61306-3.

MTA Cooperative Group (2004) National Institute of Mental Health Multimodal Treatment Study of ADHD follow-up: changes in effectiveness and growth after the end of treatment. *Pediatrics* 113: 762–769.

NICE (2008) *Attention deficit hyperactivity disorder: diagnosis and management. NICE Guidelines* [CG72], https://www.nice.org.uk/guidance/cg72.

Poulton A (2005) Growth on stimulant medication; clarifying the confusion: A review. *Arch Dis Child* 90(8): 801–806, doi:10.1136/adc.2004.056952.

Safer DJ, Allen RP, Barr E (1972) Depression of growth in hyperactive children with stimulant drugs. *N Engl J Med* 287: 217–220, doi:10.1056/NEJM197208032870503.

Sonuga-Barke EJS, Brandeis D, Cortese S et al. and the European ADHD Guidelines Group (2013) Nonpharmacological interventions for ADHD: systematic review and meta-analyses of randomized controlled trials of dietary and psychological treatments. *Am J Psychiatry* 170(3): 275–289, doi:10.1176/appi.ajp.2012.12070991.

Swanson JM, Elliott GR, Greenhill LL et al. (2007) Effect of stimulant medication on growth rates across 3 years in the MTA follow-up. *J Am Acad Child Adolesc Psychiatry* 46(8): 1015–1027, doi:10.1097/chi.0b013e3180686d7e.

Vitiello B (2008) Understanding the risk of using medications for ADHD with respect to physical growth and cardiovascular function. *Child Adolesc Psychiatr Clin N Am* 17(2): 459–xi, doi:10.1016/j.chc.2007.11.010.

Chapter 9

Cardiac issues: initial assessment and monitoring of medication

Eric Rosenthal

Case scenario

This relates to Jamie, who we met in Chapter 3, and is written by Jamie's paediatrician.

Hi,

Can I run concerns around Jamie past you?

He is 8, at private school in a small class with very good school support. You will remember his Dad was diagnosed with HOCM (hypertrophic obstructive cardiomyopathy) recently. This was causing shortness of breath and reduced exercise tolerance.

The gene testing on Dad was inconclusive. Jamie was started on EQUASYM XL He has mixed developmental difficulties/language/mild general and some specific learning difficulties alongside ADHD. Initially we were unsure medication was sufficiently effective so stopped it. However, after restarting, there has been a very, very positive impact with Jamie being much more attentive, far less confrontational. School also commented on massive improvement. Jamie was observed in school by an ADHD specialist nurse and seemed a much happier little boy producing much more work. We were initially advised not to use medication following Jamie's father's diagnosis and now are being told it is a 'judgement call'.

Jamie's ECG and echo were normal 6 months ago and I am repeating them now. I am also arranging Qb [quantitative behaviour test] on and off meds.

I also think as Jamie gets older there are now ethical issues that have not been discussed with him.

(Jamie's paediatrician)

This was followed by the following, from Jamie's father.

Dear Dr,

Firstly can I thank you for all the time and effort you have put into Jamie's case, I know it isn't straightforward.

I am writing this to let you know my thoughts about Jamie, his diagnosis of ADHD, medication and my diagnosis of HOCM. I know you had a long conversation with Kate on the phone last week and your decision to stop Jamie's medication based on your perceived balance of risks.

When we first came to your clinic I don't think Kate or I really felt that Jamie fitted into our perception of ADHD. Over the last couple of years we have come to recognise the significant ADHD traits within Jamie, particularly his inattention and impulsivity.

His inattention has caused a significant impact on his ability to learn in school, contributing to him working as a Y2 in Y5, although we realise his complex development disorder also affects his ability to learn, which includes dyspraxia, dyslexia, speech and language difficulties and a significant difficulty with numbers.

With regards to his impulsivity he is often a danger to himself, crossing roads without looking and certainly not following instructions to stop and wait for adult supervision, and generally incapable of listening to instructions.

Though we didn't think initially that medication dramatically helped Jamie we have realised over the last few months that it certainly does. This is based on the fact that his school report is very encouraging in terms of his application and engagement in all school activities. We have had a parents' evening at school last week which has confirmed the improvement in Jamie's concentration and academic progress since starting methylphenidate, finally enabling Jamie to access some of his education, and to start to make friendships with his peers, during years at school he will never be able to reclaim.

Also we have noticed over Christmas without medication, especially during the first week when he was probably tired at the end of term, that the oppositional and confrontational behaviour was markedly worsened. This made family dynamics very challenging considering we also had an emotional and exhausted 11-year-old and a 7-year-old who has modelled some behaviour on his older brother! It got to the point where I commented to Kate that I felt Jamie's behaviour was worse than it ever had been before we even started medication. Perhaps I'd just forgotten!

We are aware of family breakdowns and difficulties for siblings for those living with ADHD, and fear we could become one of those families.

Jamie is a beautiful child for so very many reasons, but asking Jamie to do the slightest thing off medication, that he may not anticipate, will lead to a red mist, and we are living in an unpleasant heightened emotional state much of the time, with Jamie being violent to his brothers and often to Kate which is taking its toll on us all.

Finally there is the news that his Qb test was startling in the improvement in his attention on medication.

I understand your dilemma about continuing medication for Jamie and your discussion with an expert at a conference. Was the expert aware about the relatively mild nature of my HOCM?

It doesn't seem to be at all severe as far as cardiologists classify it.

Then there is the issue that there is no recognised genetic marker for my HOCM which though no way conclusive, must diminish the possibility that I have an inheritable form of the condition.

In conclusion I feel that my HOCM needs to not be overemphasised in your decision making for Jamie. I feel that as medication seems clearly to be benefitting him now, and the whole family dynamics, then it is in his best interests to continue it especially in the absence of any ECG or echocardiographic abnormalities. I am asking you to consider not worrying unduly about the very slight potential for life threatening risks in the future. Of course should anything appear on surveillance, or if Jamie developed symptoms, we'd need to reconsider and probably all agree that medication should cease.

Please feel free to contact me to discuss this. I would certainly value the opportunity to discuss Jamie further before the final decision is taken on whether to discontinue Ritalin.

Many thanks to you and all the staff for your continued support of Jamie and us.

Best wishes

Jamie's Dad

Background

Medication for ADHD is most commonly with drugs that stimulate the sympathetic nervous system by various mechanisms. These include methylphenidate (release of catecholamines), amfetamines (release of catecholamines, inhibition of catecholamine and dopamine reuptake), which are grouped together as 'stimulant medications', and atomoxetine (inhibition of catecholamine reuptake), which is described as a non-stimulant. Small increases in systolic and diastolic blood pressure and heart rate are invariably reported with the use of stimulant medications and atomoxetine (Box 9.1). Usually, the rise in blood pressure is not to a level that gives clinical concern, and the mild tachycardia is rarely symptomatic. Monitoring of the pulse and blood pressure after commencement of treatment and intermittently during follow-up has been a recommendation for many years, but no further cardiac tests were advised previously (Gutgesell et al. 1999). Deaths in patients taking stimulant medications were reported infrequently except when stimulants were taken in large doses, used as a recreational drug or combined with alcohol and/or other recreational drugs.

> **Box 9.1:** Summary
>
> ✓ Methylphenidate, amfetamines and atomoxetine 'stimulate' the sympathetic system.
> ✓ A small rise in the pulse rate and blood pressure usually occurs with stimulant medication.
> ✓ Large population studies have **not** shown an increase in cardiovascular morbidity or mortality in users of stimulant medication.

The sympathomimetic effects, however, have given rise to the concept that cardiac arrhythmias and sudden cardiac death might be a cause of death in patients on stimulants. The initial case reports of sudden deaths in stimulant users and uncontrolled studies were of borderline significance, yet when this sensitive issue was raised, it caused major anxiety in the parents of children on the medication, and also prescribers. Medical and regulatory authorities reacted and led calls for 'cardiac assessment' before commencing stimulant medication in order to identify underlying cardiovascular conditions that might react badly to the administration of stimulant medication, even though there was little evidence to back this up (Nissen 2006; Conway et al. 2008). A call for an electrocardiogram (ECG) to be performed as routine before administration of stimulants was an additional contentious response (Vetter et al. 2008; Perrin et al. 2008). Further analysis of the emerging data, however, was less concerning, and large population studies subsequently showed no obvious difference in cardiovascular mortality or morbidity between current users, past users and non-users of stimulant medication (Cooper et al. 2011; Schelleman et al. 2011; Winterstein et al. 2012). Nevertheless, the genie was out the bottle, and cardiac screening and monitoring became accepted practice. The aim of such screening was to identify congenital or familial cardiovascular disorders, allowing them to be managed in their own right before commencement of stimulant medication (https://www.nice.org.uk/guidance/cg72/chapter/guidance#treatment-for-children-and-young-people; https://www.gov.uk/drug-safety-update/methylphenidate-safe-and-effective-use-to-treat-adhd; Graham et al. 2011; Hamilton et al. 2011). Very few of these congenital or familial conditions, however, would actually preclude the use of stimulants (Vetter et al. 2008; Graham et al. 2011; Hamilton et al. 2011; Rohatgi et al. 2015).

Initial history taking

History taking may elicit previous cardiac problems, a family history of heart disease or possible cardiac symptoms (Box 9.2). The history taking should seek to establish if any of the following are present:

• *Previously diagnosed congenital heart disease or prior cardiac surgery*. It is important to establish that the cardiac condition is being monitored appropriately.

A history of heart disease or of a family history of conditions associated with sudden death or cardiac symptoms indicates the need to refer a child to a paediatric cardiologist – **but** this applies to all children with these features and not just those who are about to be treated for ADHD.

- *Family history* of cardiomyopathy (hypertrophic, dilated, restrictive or undefined), channelopathy [long QT syndrome, Brugada syndrome or catecholaminergic polymorphic ventricular tachycardia (CPVT)] or sudden death in a first-degree relative under the age of 40 years could suggest a familial condition, and evaluation of *all* first-degree relatives is required (not just those being 'screened' for ADHD treatment).

- *Shortness of breath* on exertion or exercise intolerance when compared to peers may be a sign of a reduced cardiac output in children with known heart disease. It is less commonly due to an undiagnosed cardiac condition but does merit further evaluation.

- *Palpitations* that are described as fleeting skips and bumps are usually due to extra (ectopic) beats, which are common and benign and do not need investigating except in some individuals who are highly symptomatic. Rapid regular palpitations that start and stop suddenly are usually due to a supraventricular tachycardia (SVT) or, less commonly, a benign ventricular tachycardia and require further evaluation and treatment.

- *Syncope* is very common in children – perhaps in as many as one in five at some point in childhood, and is usually due to vasovagal syncope (common or benign syncope) and does not need any treatment. Certain features are suggestive of an underlying heart condition and these need further investigation. These include fainting on exertion, in response to fright or noise, when supine or with a family history of sudden death.

- *Chest pain* – this is very rarely due to the heart in children, unlike in adults. The common forms in children include a 'catch pain' that occurs on inspiration and tenderness over the chest, commonly of the costochondral junctions. Reassurance is all that is needed. A clear relationship to exercise is uncommon in children but when present should be investigated further, although it is exceedingly rare for it to be due to cardiac ischaemia and is invariably benign.

Physical examination

Before medication is prescribed, baseline pulse and blood pressure should be recorded both as normal practice but also to allow for comparison when medication is used (Box 9.3). Appendix 2 gives the correct cuff sizes for measuring blood pressure and the normal

> **Box 9.3:** Physical examination
>
> ✓ Physical findings suggestive of cardiac disease indicate the need to refer a child to a paediatric cardiologist – but this applies to all children with these features and not just those who are about to be treated for ADHD.
> ✓ A persistently raised BP indicates the need to refer to a paediatric hypertension specialist for further evaluation.
> ✓ A baseline BP & pulse rate are used to compare any changes occurring during stimulant treatment.

range for blood pressure measurements adjusted for height, age and sex. Appendix 3 lists normal pulse rate ranges.

Look for signs of undiagnosed heart disease
• *Signs of heart failure:* breathlessness, pallor and sweating at rest, tachycardia, gallop rhythm on auscultation, ankle oedema and hepatomegaly.

• *Cyanosis:* indicating undiagnosed cyanotic heart disease (extremely rare).

• *Murmurs:* although the majority are benign (normal or innocent), mild forms of congenital heart disease may be first identified in older children.

• *Absent or weak femoral pulses* may be due to an undiagnosed coarctation of the aorta (usually with raised arm blood pressure and a murmur).

The presence of any of these merits referral to a paediatric cardiologist.

Monitoring of stimulant medication
At every monitoring visit, blood pressure and pulse should be measured and checked against normal values for age, sex and height (Appendices 2 and 3). If the child/young person reports any of the symptoms stated in the initial history, consider further assessment at any point.

Electrocardiogram

An ECG is able to detect some forms of heart disease that are not apparent on a history or physical examination and often confirms findings suggestive of cardiac disease in the history or examination (Box 9.4). Not all cardiac diseases are detectable with an ECG, and some that are may be present only intermittently or become apparent at different ages. There is controversy as to whether ECG screening should be offered before sports

---

Box 9.4: ECG

✓ A normal ECG does not exclude many forms of heart disease.

✓ Many variants of normal on an ECG may cause unnecessary alarm to non-specialists, especially when a 'computer diagnosis' is based on an adult algorithm.

✓ An ECG should *not* be used for 'screening' prior to commencing stimulant medication in ADHD.

✓ An ECG *should* be obtained before administration of tricyclic antidepressants and mono amine oxidase inhibitors and other agents that affect the QT interval.

---

participation and the same applies to screening before ADHD medication. A move to offer ECG screening to all children has been debated for several years. Constraints would include the low sensitivity for all cardiac disease, low specificity with a number of normal variants that confuse non-experts, and lack of an infrastructure to deliver such a programme. In addition, it is not clear whether such an expensive undertaking should be performed at several ages in childhood to detect evolving conditions.

An ECG is *not needed* before commencing stimulant medication in a child who has had a clinical evaluation as part of the initial history and clinical examination (Perrin et al. 2008; https://www.nice.org.uk/guidance/cg72/chapter/guidance#treatment-for-children-and-young-people; Graham et al. 2011; Hamilton et al. 2011).

An ECG is, however, mandatory before the administration of medications that affect the QT interval (tricyclic antidepressants and mono amine oxidase inhibitors) to establish a baseline and for serial evaluation as the doses are changed or additional agents are used (Gutgesell et al.1999; Vetter et al. 2008).

When to refer to a cardiologist

When there are features in either the history or examination that are suggestive of cardiac disease, a referral to a paediatric cardiologist is appropriate. This would apply to the same findings in a child being seen for another issue or symptom and is not specific to 'screening' for ADHD or before participation for sports. At this stage, the cardiologist can perform an ECG, an echocardiogram and any other appropriate tests as needed.

When to refer to a blood pressure specialist

When there is elevation of the blood pressure (above the 95th centile for age and height) at baseline that persists.

Measurement of blood pressure away from the clinic (e.g. at school) is essential to ensure the child is not simply anxious at the clinic. It is also easy to check the urine for blood, protein or infection. Referral to a paediatric hypertension specialist (commonly a paediatrician or nephrologist rather than a cardiologist) is then required. Further blood pressure assessment and investigations for an underlying cause can be instigated at that stage if appropriate. Full evaluation of primary and secondary hypertension is described in 'The Fourth Report on the Diagnosis, Evaluation, and Treatment of High Blood Pressure in Children and Adolescents' (NIH 1996/2015).

Ongoing monitoring

Blood pressure
The small rise in blood pressure is not considered to be clinically significant in the majority of children on stimulant treatment. In some with borderline blood pressure before treatment, even a small increase may take them above the 95th centile, while in some the absolute rise is more significant and they also increase to above the 95th centile. First, it is appropriate to check the blood pressure off medication and away from the clinic setting. A 24-hour blood pressure monitoring tape can also be helpful as a blood pressure that returns to normal during sleep is reassuring. If the blood pressure remains elevated, referral to a hypertension specialist is required to discuss the need for further investigation (e.g. renal function testing, renal ultrasound, etc.), and reduction or cessation of stimulant treatment or addition of antihypertensive medication while continuing stimulant medication according to the needs of the patient. If a consistent and significant rise in blood pressure occurs but the absolute value does not go above the 95th centile, there is no need to stop or reduce medication if this is otherwise optimal for the individual child. However, monitoring at 3 months, perhaps by the general practitioner (GP) or in school, would be appropriate as a further rise may occur.

The consensus is that 6-monthly blood pressure estimations in the first few years of treatment are good practice, although the frequency could be reduced to yearly if normal blood pressure is maintained (https://www.nice.org.uk/guidance/cg72/chapter/guidance#treatment-for-children-and-young-people; Graham et al. 2011; Hamilton et al. 2011).

Heart rate
In some children, the rise in heart rate appears to be more than a few beats per minute and they may be aware of this. This should be distinguished from non-medication-related ectopics or sustained intermittent tachycardias (see section 'Initial history taking').

Reduction in the dose or a change in the formulation may be helpful. A 24-hour tape recording may be very helpful in clarifying diagnosis. Rarely, medication to reduce this side effect (e.g. a beta-blocker) might be needed. Unless the heart rate is persistently above 120 beats per minute it is unlikely to have any effects on heart function over the long term.

Do not assume medication is to blame.

Always remember that raised blood pressure or pulse may also be due to completely separate causes, not the medication (e.g. renal problems or hyperthyroidism).

Children who develop effort intolerance, palpitations, syncope or chest pain on exertion during follow-up will require a cardiology referral (see section 'When to refer to a cardiologist') as would any child with these symptoms unrelated to the diagnosis of ADHD or use of stimulant medication.

When is stimulant medication not advised?

There are very few children who are unable to take stimulant medication due to their underlying cardiovascular condition. The NICE guidelines suggest that groups with the following conditions should NOT receive stimulants UNLESS discussed with a paediatric cardiologist:

- haemodynamically significant congenital heart disease

- heart failure

- cardiomyopathies

- potentially life-threatening arrhythmias

- dysfunction of cardiac ion channels (channelopathies)

- arterial occlusive disease and angina and myocardial infarction (rare in children)

- severe hypertension

In practice, very few of these would not be eligible once the ADHD specialist, paediatric cardiologist and family or patient have considered the issues (Vetter et al. 2008; Graham et al. 2011; Hamilton et al. 2011). Indeed, even the long QT syndrome that, per se, carries a risk of sudden death is not an absolute contra-indication to stimulant medication when all the issues are considered – severity of ADHD, severity of long QT syndrome, medication for long QT syndrome, use of implantable defibrillators and the family and patient attitude to risk (Rohatgi et al. 2015; Zhang et al. 2015).

Case scenarios

It should now be possible to consider some possible scenarios.

Michael, a 12-year-old boy with ADHD, was being considered for treatment with methylphenidate. The family history and clinical examination were unremarkable with a blood pressure in the normal range. An ECG was performed 'as screening before medication' and the computer diagnosis was of 'incomplete right bundle branch block, borderline prolonged QT interval; abnormal ECG'. The methylphenidate was not commenced. Several months later, after major behavioural difficulties at home and at school, the ECG was shown to a paediatric cardiologist. Incomplete right bundle branch block is a normal variant and was ignored. Manual measurement of the QT interval and calculation of the QTc showed this to be at the upper end of the normal range. Management had therefore been based on an unvalidated 'computer diagnosis' that was incorrect. Methylphenidate was prescribed for Michael, with a major improvement in core ADHD symptoms, which then improved his behaviour. Michael and his family were very pleased this had been resolved. No further cardiac investigations were indicated.

Learning point: In a child with no family history of a channelopathy, cardiomyopathy or sudden death at a young age, no history of cardiac disease or cardiac symptoms and a normal physical examination, the ECG adds little to the assessment of suitability for stimulant medication (and needs to be interpreted correctly IF performed). Our view is that it is better NOT to perform an ECG in this setting.

Jimmy, a 10-year-old boy with ADHD, was found to have a significant cardiac murmur. He was an active child with good exercise tolerance and no signs of heart failure. Methylphenidate was not commenced and he was referred to a paediatric cardiologist. An echocardiogram showed a secundum atrial septal defect (ASD) that was large enough to merit closure. The cardiologist recommended that methylphenidate could be commenced immediately and closure of J's ASD could be performed as a routine procedure in the next 3–6 months after the family's planned holiday trip.

Learning point: Any child in whom an abnormal history or physical examination indicates cardiac disease should be seen by a paediatric cardiologist – irrespective of whether he has ADHD or whether medication is being considered. In this patient, a new diagnosis of congenital heart disease was made, allowing appropriate treatment. It was also a condition that did not preclude stimulant therapy either before or after treatment. Ongoing cardiac management and ADHD treatment could therefore proceed independently.

Becky, a 13-year-old girl with severe symptoms of ADHD, was being considered for stimulant treatment. Her father had died suddenly at the age of 36 years, with a normal post-mortem examination. There were no cardiac symptoms or abnormal findings on examination. In view of the family history, she was referred to a paediatric cardiologist. The cardiologist found her to have a mildly prolonged QT interval (475ms), which, in the context of the family history, was considered to be important. Genetic testing revealed she was a carrier of a long QT I gene abnormality and all her first-degree relatives were therefore enrolled for screening. She was commenced on a beta-blocker for prevention of sudden death. Prescription of stimulant medication was considered. It is recognised that certain medications can provoke arrhythmias and sudden death in long QT patients, in spite of appropriate beta-blocker treatment. The long QT syndrome list of drugs to avoid includes the stimulant medications (http://www.sads.org. uk/drugs_to_avoid.htm) and at first glance these would have been contraindicated in Becky. However, given the severity of her ADHD symptoms, the mildly prolonged QT interval and adherence to beta-blockers, it was felt that the administration of stimulants at as low a dose as possible with regular cardiac monitoring was appropriate.

Learning point: Any child with a family history of arrhythmic sudden death should be seen by a paediatric cardiologist, irrespective of whether he/she has ADHD or whether medication is being considered. The diagnosis of long QT syndrome allowed screening of first-degree relatives and treatment of the condition in the child. The decision to use stimulant therapy could only be made after careful consideration of the child by the ADHD specialist, cardiologist and the family. In this child, a balanced decision was made to allow stimulant treatment after discussions between the family and the specialists (Graham et al. 2011; Hamilton et al. 2011; Rohatgi et al. 2015; Zhang et al. 2015).

Summary

- History taking should include past history of cardiac disease or surgery, possible symptoms of cardiovascular disease and family history of cardiac problems or sudden death under the age of 40 years.

- Presence of any of these merits referral to a cardiologist.

- Children without any of these do not need ECG before the use of medication.

- If new information or symptoms occur during monitoring, refer then.

- Raised blood pressure (>95th centile) at baseline or on monitoring merits referral to a specialist.

- Provided monitoring is in place, most children and young people with ADHD can take medication.

References

Conway J, Wong KK, O'Connell C, Warren AE (2008) Cardiovascular risk screening before starting stimulant medications and prescribing practices of Canadian physicians: Impact of the Health Canada Advisory. *Pediatrics* 122: e828–e834.

Cooper WO, Habel LA, Sox CM et al. (2011) ADHD drugs and serious cardiovascular events in children and young adults. *N Engl J Med* 365: 1896–1904.

Gutgesell H, Atkins D, Barst R et al. (1999) Cardiovascular monitoring of children and adolescents receiving psychotropic drugs: A statement for healthcare professionals from the Committee on Congenital Cardiac Defects, Council on Cardiovascular Disease in the Young, American Heart Association. *Circulation* 99: 979–982.

Graham J, Banaschewski T, Buitelaar J et al. (2011) European guidelines on managing adverse effects of medication for ADHD. *Eur Child Adolesc Psychiatry* 20: 17–37.

Hamilton RM, Rosenthal E, Hulpke-Wette M, Graham JG, Sergeant J (2011) Cardiovascular considerations of attention deficit hyperactivity disorder medications: A report of the European Network on Hyperactivity Disorders work group, European Attention Deficit Hyperactivity Disorder Guidelines Group on attention deficit hyperactivity disorder drug safety meeting. *Cardiol Young* 19: 1–8, 17.

NICE (2009) https://www.gov.uk/drug-safety-update/methylphenidate-safe-and-effective-use-to-treat-adhd.

NIH (1996/2005) *The Fourth Report on the diagnosis, evaluation, and treatment of high blood pressure in children and adolescents*, NIH Publication No. 05-5267. Bethesday, MD: US Department of Health and Human Services, National Institutes of Health National Heart, Lung, and Blood Institute.

Nissen SE (2006) ADHD drugs and cardiovascular risk. *N Engl J Med* 354: 1445–1448.

Perrin JM, Friedman RA, Knilans TK and the Black Box Working Group, Section on Cardiology and Cardiac Surgery (2008) Cardiovascular monitoring and stimulant drugs for attention-deficit/hyperactivity disorder. *Pediatrics* 122(2): 451–453, doi:10.1542/peds.2008-1573.

Rohatgi RK, Bos JM, Ackerman MJ (2015) Stimulant therapy in children with attention-deficit/hyperactivity disorder and concomitant long QT syndrome: A safe combination? *Heart Rhythm* 12(8): 1807–1812, doi:10.1016/j.hrthm.2015.04.043.

Schelleman H, Bilker WB, Strom BL et al. (2011) Cardiovascular events and death in children exposed and unexposed to ADHD agents. *Pediatrics* 127(6): 1102–1110.

Vetter VL, Elia J, Erickson C et al. (2008) Cardiovascular monitoring of children and adolescents with heart disease receiving medications for attention deficit/hyperactivity disorder [corrected]: a scientific statement from the American Heart Association Council on Cardiovascular Disease in the Young Congenital Cardiac Defects Committee and the Council on Cardiovascular Nursing. *Circulation* 117: 2407–2423.

Winterstein AG, Gerhard T, Kubilis P et al. (2012) Cardiovascular safety of central nervous system stimulants in children and adolescents: Population based cohort study. *BMJ* 345: e4627.

Zhang C, Kutyifa V, Moss AJ, McNitt S, Zareba W, Kaufman ES (2015) Long-QT syndrome and therapy for attention deficit/hyperactivity disorder. *J Cardiovasc Electrophysiol* 26(10): 1039–1044, doi:10.1111/jce.12739.

Chapter 10

School and classroom strategies for the teaching and management of children with ADHD

Fintan O'Regan

School will provide a number of challenges for children with ADHD, their teachers, their peers and for the parents/carers of the child concerned. This chapter considers some of the options available to increase the likelihood of successful outcomes in school, with particular reference to the UK.

The impact of a child with ADHD on both the classroom and non-classroom time within a school community should not be underestimated, but there can be many positives as well as challenges. The key is both to acknowledge the specific learning, behavioural and socialisation needs of each child and then to adapt systems and strategies to meet those needs and develop strengths further.

The question is sometimes asked whether children with ADHD should be included within the mainstream school system or placed within special schools. As with any other child with special needs, all children with ADHD should be assessed individually, and appropriate support to meet their needs should be provided, initially in a mainstream setting. Evaluation should determine the level of learning, behavioural and socialisation needed. Comorbid developmental difficulties also need to be taken into account, and specific strategies for these implemented. If evaluation and ongoing monitoring demonstrate greater needs, then special schooling should be considered to optimise learning.

Teaching children with ADHD

Teaching and managing children with ADHD can be summed up in three main words: *structure*, *flexibility* and *relationships*. Having said this, there are some tried and tested strategies that may well help support specific individuals at specific times during the day. Some of the following suggestions will not work for everyone, but the key is not what you do but *how* you do it.

Initial strategies to be employed in classroom practice

When a child or young person with ADHD is in a school setting, a number of management strategies should be put in place immediately. These include the following:

- Seat the student near to the teacher with his/her back to the rest of the class to keep other students out of view.

- Surround the student with good role models, preferably those seen as 'significant others': facilitate peer tutoring and cooperative learning.

- Avoid distracting stimuli. Place the learners away from heaters/air conditioners, doors or windows, high-traffic areas and computers.

- Children and young people with ADHD do not handle change well, so minimise changes in schedule, physical relocation and disruptions, and give plenty of warning when changes are about to occur.

- Create a 'stimuli reduced area' for all students to access. Using this should not be seen as a punishment if things go wrong, but as a positive choice to help.

- Maintain eye contact with student during verbal instruction, and avoid multiple commands/requests.

- Make directions clear and concise. Be consistent with daily instructions and expectations.

- Give one task at a time, but monitor frequently.

- Make sure the student understands before beginning the task, and repeat the explanation in a calm, positive manner, if needed.

- Help the child or young person to feel comfortable with seeking assistance (most learners with ADHD will not ask).

- A child with ADHD may need more help for a longer period of time than the average child. As time goes on, reduce assistance gradually.

- Use a day-book. Make sure the student writes down assignments and that both parents and teachers sign the book daily to show they have seen homework tasks.

- Modify assignments as necessary, developing an individualised programme and allowing extra time when appropriate.

- Make sure you are testing knowledge and not attention span.

Once the structure has been established, then flexibility in terms of learning can take place. Many children with ADHD are likely to be very weak in a host of fundamental areas. Some of the following suggestions will help in supporting their development of basic skills.

English skills and reading comprehension

- *Partner reading activities*. Pair the child with ADHD with another student partner who is a strong reader. The partners take turns reading orally and listening to each other.

- *Play-acting*. Schedule play-acting sessions where the child can role-play different characters.

- *Word bank*. Keep a word bank or dictionary of new or hard-to-sight-read vocabulary words.

- *Board games for reading comprehension*. Play board games that provide practice with target reading-comprehension skills or sight vocabulary words.

- *Computer games for reading comprehension*. Schedule computer time for the child to have drill-and-practice with sight vocabulary words.

- *Recorded books*. These materials can stimulate interest in reading and increase a child's confidence.

- *Backup materials for home use*. Make available a second set of books and materials that can be used at home.

- *Summary materials*. Allow and encourage students to use published book summaries, synopses and digests of major reading assignments to review (not replace) reading assignments.

Phonics

To help children with ADHD master the rules of phonics, the following are effective:

- *Mnemonics for phonics*. Teach the child mnemonics that provide reminders about hard-to-learn phonics rules (e.g. 'when two vowels go walking, the first does the talking').

- *Computer games for phonics.* Use a computer to provide opportunities for drill and practice.

Writing

Many children with ADHD also have motor coordination difficulties that add to their problems with recording their work. In composing stories or other writing assignments, children with ADHD benefit from the following practices:

- *Standards for writing assignments.* Identify and teach the child classroom standards for acceptable written work, such as format and style.

- *Recognising parts of a story.* Teach the student how to describe the major parts of a story (e.g. plot, main characters, setting, conflict and resolution).

- *Proofread completed work.* Provide the student with a list of items to check when proofreading his or her own work, or swap with a 'critical friend'.

- *Recording.* Ask the student to dictate writing assignments into a recorder, or use voice recognition software as an alternative to writing.

- *Dictate writing assignments.* Have the teacher or another student write down a story told by a child with ADHD.

Spelling

To help children with ADHD who are poor spellers, the following techniques have been found to be helpful:

- *Everyday examples of hard-to-spell words.* Take advantage of everyday events to teach spellings in context. For example, for a child who is quite confrontational in class, look at words like 'compromise', 'concede' and 'acquiesce'.

- *Frequently used words.* For learning/testing spellings, assign words that the child routinely uses in his or her speech each day.

- *Dictionary of misspelled words.* Ask the child to keep a personal dictionary of frequently misspelled words.

- *Partner spelling activities.* Pair the child with another student. Ask the partners to quiz each other on the spelling of new words. Encourage both students to guess the correct spelling.

- *Colour-coded letters.* Colour code different letters in hard-to-spell words (e.g. 'receipt').

- *Word banks.* Use index cards to store frequently misspelled words sorted alphabetically, or an alphabet sheet (A4, with boxes for words starting with each letter of the alphabet).

Maths

Numerous individualised instructional practices can help children and young people with ADHD improve their basic computation skills. The following are just a few:

- *Partnering for maths activities.* Pair the student with ADHD with another student and provide opportunities for the partners to quiz each other about basic computation skills.

- *Language of maths.* If the child or young person does not understand the symbols and language used in maths, they will not be able to do the work. For instance, do they understand terms such as 'product' and 'quotient'? Provide a maths dictionary or bank of key words.

- *Mnemonics for basic computation.* Teach mnemonics that describe basic steps in computing whole numbers. For example:

  'Don't Miss Susie's Boat' can be used to help the student recall the basic steps in long division (i.e. divide, multiply, subtract and bring down);

  SOCA for Sine–Opposite, Cosine–Adjacent.

- *Real-life examples of money skills.* Provide real-life opportunities to practise target money skills. For example, ask the student to calculate his or her change when paying for lunch in the school cafeteria, or set up a class store where all students can practise calculating change. (Plastic money is fine for younger children but use real coins for older students if they are unable to deal in the abstract.)

- *Calculators to check basic computation.* Ask the child or young person to use a calculator to check addition, subtraction, multiplication or division.

- *Board games for basic computation.* Ask the student with ADHD to play board games to practice skills (such as Othello or Connect 4).

- *Computer games for basic computation.* Schedule computer time to practise basic computations, using appropriate games.

Depending on the pupil's level of literacy and numeracy development, the support of a teaching assistant may be appropriate, or tuition from a specialist dyslexia teacher. In these circumstances, it is important that the adult involved is familiar with the student's specific needs regarding ADHD, as well as the literacy/numeracy targets. Consistency between the classroom/class teacher and other adults involved with the child or young person is paramount.

Technology

Materials used may vary according to the techniques employed, but should always be as attractive and engaging as possible, as well as age-appropriate. There is no doubt that many approaches involve IT (information technology), which appears to be a medium that relates well to the learning processes of children with ADHD for a number of reasons (Box 10.1). Literacy and spelling programmes such as the Active Literacy Kit (and especially Units of Sound) appear particularly effective, along with Word Shark, Number Shark, Text Detective and a host of others in the market.

Help with study skills for students with ADHD

Children and young people with ADHD often have difficulty in learning how to study effectively on their own. The following strategies may assist them in developing the skills necessary for academic success:

- *Adapt worksheets*. Teach the student how to adapt instructional worksheets so that they do not seem overwhelming. For example, fold the worksheet to reveal only one question at a time, or use a piece of card or a ruler.

- *Venn diagrams*. Teach how to use Venn diagrams to help illustrate and organise key concepts or pieces of information in a particular topic.

- *Note-taking skills*. Teach a student with ADHD how to take notes when organising key concepts that he or she has learned, perhaps with the use of a program such as Anita Archer's Skills for School Success.

- *Checklist of frequent mistakes*. Provide a checklist of mistakes that the student makes frequently in written assignments (e.g. punctuation or capitalisation errors), mathematics (e.g. addition or subtraction errors) or other academic subjects.

Box 10.1: Reasons why using IT is helpful to students with ADHD

✓ The child responds well to an individualised or one-to-one setting
✓ Attention is focused on the screen
✓ Technology provides multisensory experiences
✓ Computers are non-threatening and provide constant feedback and reinforcement
✓ A computer is impersonal – it doesn't yell or have favourites
✓ A variety of presentation styles ensures better attention
✓ Students can control the pace and 'try again' if necessary
✓ Computers are flexible in that they can be programmed to do many things
✓ Students can receive rapid assessment
✓ A game-like approach appeals to pupils with ADHD and they enjoy the challenge

Teach the student how to use this list when proofreading his or her work at home and school.

- *Uncluttered workspace*. Teach a child or young person with ADHD how to prepare an uncluttered workspace to complete assignments. For example, instruct them to clear away unnecessary books or other materials before beginning his or her classwork.

- *Monitor homework assignments*. Keep track of how well your students with ADHD complete their assigned homework. Discuss and resolve, with them and their parents, any problems in completing these assignments. For example, evaluate the difficulty of the assignments and how long the student spends on their homework each night.

Homework

The considered opinion is that it takes a pupil with ADHD at least three times as long to do a piece of work at home as it would take to do in school. The many distractions of home and a more casual, unstructured environment mean that attention is less focused and therefore everything takes longer. It may be better for the child to do homework in a homework club if possible; however, if this is not possible, then offer parents advice (Box 10.2).

With the time element in mind, teachers should differentiate homework to ensure that pupils with ADHD do not have to spend three times as long as peers on any given assignment. This is very discouraging and in the long run counter-productive.

Flexibility should extend beyond homework to other aspects of school life including test taking and examinations.

Box 10.2: Advice to parents about homework

✓ Monitor homework set each day
✓ Ask your child to explain what he/she has to do
✓ Establish a routine time for the completion of homework (e.g. after tea, before the television or games console is switched on)
✓ Minimise distractions (e.g. younger siblings)
✓ Provide a clear surface in a quiet space

and

✓ Always take an interest

For Key Stage and GCSE examinations, a whole host of special arrangements exist for students with a range of special needs including ADHD. It is important that teachers know about all of the possibilities and how and when to apply for them. Practice in advance is also an essential requirement for success, for example working with a reader (amanuensis) is a skilled technique and students will need to have a number of trials before attempting the examination. Current special arrangement options are listed in Box 10.3.

Behaviour management

One of the most difficult parts of managing students with ADHD is the issue of avoiding and dealing with disruptions in the classroom. One effective technique involves the use of non-verbal direction. Most direction by teachers is done through verbal instructions, but research has shown that non-verbal direction can be much more effective for children with ADHD (Geng 2011).

General advice in terms of reducing disruption and improving attention is to use your own presence by moving near to the child on occasions that you think warrant this approach. Simply standing close behind or beside the child can often dampen the activity level of an individual to dramatic effect without a word being spoken about the student's behaviour. Tactical ignoring of attention-seeking behaviour is another option, with a 'knowing look' or a shake of the head making it clear that this is not acceptable sometimes being enough. If only you or a few students appear affected by actions that are more covert, a quick tap on the shoulder and a word in the ear that you will catch up with them later may be enough.

If the actions are more disruptive and affecting the whole class, meet the situation with a firm but business-like approach, saying that that this behaviour is not appropriate. Give only one warning that if the behaviour is repeated there will be consequences. One warning, not two, is to be advised.

Box 10.3: Current possible special arrangement options for examinations

✓ Extra time allowance
✓ Rest periods
✓ Use of a reader
✓ Amanuensis
✓ Use of word processors
✓ Spelling, punctuation and grammar support
✓ Prompters

Finally, praise for appropriate responses will always be a welcome option. It is also worth considering involving the rest of the class in supporting a child with ADHD. Encourage them to help by not 'winding them up' or provoking them into being the class clown.

Verbal or physical aggression towards either peers or teachers warrants our full attention. Regardless of the cause, whether frustration at not learning or other experiences of being misunderstood, aggression cannot be tolerated. Reversing aggression can take a great deal of time and supervision. In some cases, the issues are multifaceted in origin and therefore will be multi-agency in management, involving some or all of the following: counsellors, peer mentors, form tutors, parents, social services and health professionals. Taking note of the timing of aggressive outbursts may be informative (e.g. if the student is on medication is this wearing off?) Also remember comorbid conditions. Anxiety or intolerance of change in a student with comorbid autism spectrum disorder may result in aggressive outbursts to avoid the situation. Always consider what happens before an outburst. This helps to put in place preventative strategies.

Aggression towards others by students with ADHD should always result in logical consequences, however. A student who exhibits this trait on a regular basis has to learn that aggression towards others will result in an immediate response from teachers, with no warnings necessary. The usual sanction is to remove the student from the classroom and place him/her in a 'time out' zone or other suitable, stimuli-free area. There are a number of time out systems, but probably the best structured approach is the 1, 2, 3 Magic system by Thomas Phelan (2016), a highly effective home and classroom behavioural modification system (Phelan & Schonour 2016).

Other options in dealing with aggression include teaching the child to use hesitation and calming techniques before the 'blue mist' gains momentum, and to find alternative ways of dealing with aggressive feelings and attitudes.

Working with parents

A key issue for all schools is to develop positive partnerships with parents in order to provide a two-way flow of information, knowledge and expertise, and this is especially important for families with children and adolescents who have ADHD. Common features of effective practice in partnership include the following:

- School staff showing respect for the role of parents in their child's education: recognising and acknowledging the part they play in teaching values and shaping behaviour.

- Encouragement for parents to actively support their child's education.

- Staff who listen to parents' accounts of their children's development and take action to address concerns they may have.

- Ensuring that parents feel welcome, valued and necessary through a range of different opportunities for collaboration between children, parents and practitioners, even when things become very difficult.

- Keeping parents informed about the curriculum through the use of brochures, displays and videos, which are made available in the parents' home language.

- Regular opportunities to talk with staff and record information about progress and achievements (not just constant reports of negatives).

- Relevant school-learning opportunities being shared with home, and home experiences being valued and used to promote learning.

In some cases, parents will turn to the school, and often the Special Educational Needs Co-ordinator (SENCO), for advice about what they should be doing at home. This can be difficult to avoid, but care should be taken as difficulties can arise if strategies you suggest backfire. The best way to handle this is to direct parents towards the large amount of home management material available from support groups, such as the ADHD parent support group The National Attention Deficit Disorder Information and Support Service (ADDISS, www.addiss.co.uk).

Transitions

Moving from a less structured, more play-orientated environment in the early years to a more formalised classroom setting may both be problematic but also beneficial for children with ADHD. The open, less structured early years environment may have suited the ADHD impulsive learning style, but the potential for accidents and incidents may have already resulted in the child with ADHD acquiring a 'reputation' among teachers, peers and parents of the other children. As a result, the more structured classroom environment may provide a positive opportunity for the application of the rules, rituals and routines needed by children with ADHD.

Teacher training in both classroom and curriculum management will be vital for successful transition to take place.

However, most important of all, and most difficult to implement, is to promote the acceptance of both peers and of the parents of peers of a child who may be regarded as disruptive and difficult but who is essentially different. It is likely that some degree of social exclusion has already taken place. Many parties and sleepover invites will not have included the child with ADHD, leading to a loss of self-esteem and confidence by the individual and his family.

Wherever possible it is advised that during Personal Social Health and Economics (PSHE) lessons and Circle Time/Circle of Friends, opportunities should be taken to explore the differences of individuals within an inclusive community.

One of the most important decisions to be made about a child's education involves the choice of secondary school. For parents of a child with ADHD, this is especially challenging. They will look for a secondary school that can offer a level of understanding and continuity of structure similar to that provided by a successful primary school. However, this can be a difficult quest. Time and time again, hopes and aspirations of parents have been dashed by the huge differences that exist between primary and secondary settings. They need to be aware of what can reasonably be expected, how they can differentiate between schools and the criteria to use in making an all-important choice. The primary school SENCO has a crucial role to play in this process, ensuring that parents are well informed and able to ask appropriate questions regarding the most relevant issues. In addition to all of the usual features of schools, such as facilities, academic success, reputation and so on, the parents of a child with ADHD will also be concerned with a number of other issues (Box 10.4).

Education health and care plans

In the UK, children and young people with special educational needs that are not being met, despite appropriate input from their school, may be considered for an Education Health and Care Plan (EHCP). This involves monitoring school progress and gathering reports from relevant education-based and other professionals including Health. The majority of children with ADHD do not reach the levels of impairment that trigger an EHCP assessment, but some will, especially those with complex comorbidity or severe

---

Box 10.4: Additional qualities to look for in a secondary school for a pupil with ADHD

✓ The attitude of the head teacher and senior management team (SMT) with regards to ADHD
✓ The role, status and expertise of the secondary school SENCO (Has he/she got experience of supporting children with ADHD?)
✓ The school's arrangements for supporting children with ADHD during non-structured time
✓ How the school deals with, and helps to improve pupils' weak personal organisation
✓ How class work and homework is differentiated
✓ The school's attitude towards working with external agencies (e.g. educational psychologists, health, social services and those involved in anti-social behaviour)
✓ How the school/SENCO communicates with parents
✓ Arangements for the child to take medication (though long-acting medication formulations can provide unbroken coverage throughout the school day)

behavioural difficulties. If an assessment takes place, input will be requested from the ADHD team and other involved health professionals (e.g. autism specialists). Reports should cover information confirming diagnoses and should suggest strategies to support the child/young person. Clearly this should be discussed with the family (including the child), teachers and educational psychologists.

Summary

- Although there are many challenges in teaching and managing children with ADHD in schools, there are also many opportunities and many strengths that can be nurtured. There are techniques that will positively support the child/young person and help the teacher and others in the class.

- Thought needs to be given to classroom time and to unstructured times out of class, as both can be difficult for children/young people with ADHD.

- Through structure with flexibility, creativity, and positive relationships with children and young people with ADHD and their families, many successful outcomes can take place.

- The key is to understand the condition and to remember that fairness is not giving every child the same, but giving them what they need.

References

Geng G (2011) Investigation of teachers' verbal and non-verbal strategies for managing attention deficit hyperactivity disorder (ADHD) students' behaviours within a classroom environment. *Austral J Teacher Educ* 36(7): http://dx.doi.org/10.14221/ajte.2011v36n7.5.

Phelan T, Schonour SJ (2016) *1-2-3 magic for teachers: Effective classroom disciplines pre-K through grade 8*. Child Management Inc., Naperville, IL.

Phelan T (2016) *1-2-3 magic: Effective discipline for children 2-12*, 6th edn. Sourcebooks, Naperville, IL.

Chapter 11

How coexisting difficulties may affect the management of ADHD

Val Harpin and Shatha Shibib

I wanted to let you know we are 3 days into meds and it has literally revolutionised our life. She has just spent 20 minutes looking through recipe books looking for a pudding we can make to take to a friend's house. And she is engaging so much better in responsive conversation, following instructions and her entire body is stiller. She has read books with me without moving once. I am astounded at the impact.

(Message left by the mother of a girl with ASD, learning disability and ADHD after starting long-acting methylphenidate)

This chapter will consider how common comorbid difficulties may impact on ADHD management. As the majority of children and young people with ADHD have at least one comorbid developmental or mental health difficulty, the overall care plan must include management of these difficulties in addition to ADHD management. Sometimes, the relevant clinical expertise to assess and treat a comorbidity is present within the ADHD assessment team, but sometimes, awareness of the issues and onward referral to other clinicians is needed. Ideally, Child and Adolescent Mental Health Services (CAMHS) and paediatric teams working in a locality will develop close links so that to-and-fro referral is effective for families rather than becoming a barrier.

The order of interventions and the possible impact, positive or negative, of interventions needs to be considered. If a child or young person appears to be having a particularly challenging time it is also vital to assess the different contributions of coexisting problems and take this into account when planning support. Verbal and, if available, written information about each coexisting diagnosis should be shared with the family.

Overall, the presence of comorbid conditions appears to have an adverse effect on the response to treatment (Setyawan et al. 2015), and optimisation can be complex.

Oppositional defiant disorder

When a child is diagnosed with ADHD, all parents should be offered parent management skills training specific to children with ADHD. When given at an early stage, such skills can significantly reduce current and perhaps future oppositional defiant disorder (ODD) symptoms. Young people with ODD may also be offered therapeutic work to explore and address any underlying difficulties contributing to their behaviour.

Medication for ADHD, both stimulants and non-stimulants, frequently helps to reduce ODD symptoms (Jensen et al. 2001; Biederman et al. 2007) and has been shown to improve quality of life measures (Newcorn et al. 2005). However, higher doses are often needed to achieve improvement, and titration should take this into account.

Oppositional symptoms may also increase as a child moves into adolescence, and additional specific support should be offered to families around this time rather than necessarily increasing medication.

Conduct disorder

Children and young people with conduct disorder will need a multifaceted management plan involving health, education, social care and other statutory and voluntary services.

Early-onset conduct disorder is often related to severe family psychopathology. To support the child optimally it will be necessary to find out about relevant family issues, whether any services are involved in helping resolve these and whether any additional referrals (e.g. to Adult Mental Health) are needed. Children with severe conduct disorder alongside ADHD are often less responsive to treatment and need long-term support. If the child attends a special school or is out of school because of their behaviour, particularly close work with the school or education services is required, perhaps including clinics within school and regular multidisciplinary meetings.

In later-onset conduct disorder (>12 years of age), significant social disadvantage is frequently present. A multiagency package may help to reduce the impact of disadvantage on vulnerable young people and, for example, extremely close working with Education may help the young person remain in education, providing an increased possibility of later employment. Multisystemic therapy may be indicated for those with severe behavioural and psychosocial difficulties. This is an intensive treatment programme that is family focused, which takes place in the home and community. Evidence suggests this can be helpful to reduce conduct problems, antisocial behaviour and substance misuse (van der Stouwe et al. 2014).

Group work with these young people is potentially negative, sometimes resulting in group education on antisocial behaviour rather than how to avoid it. Referral to local Youth Services can, however, provide much needed support in the community.

The increased risk of depression in young people with ADHD and conduct disorder means that frequent review of mood is needed and, if necessary, treatment should be instigated. The involvement of a Forensic CAMHS Team and Youth Offending Team should be offered when offending has taken place or seems likely to do so.

In the presence of persistent and severe challenging behaviour, antipsychotic medication may be considered as an adjunct. If antipsychotic medication is deemed appropriate, pretreatment electrocardiogram (ECG) and blood tests (full blood count, fasting blood glucose, HbA1C, cholesterol, lipids, liver function tests and electrolytes and prolactin) will be needed, as well as careful ongoing monitoring of possible side effects (including excessive weight gain and increased blood pressure) and blood profile.

Also, this group is especially at risk of substance misuse. Early identification, psychoeducation and referral for specific treatment may be necessary (see Chapter 15).

Anxiety

When children/young people have anxiety and ADHD, consideration should be given to non-pharmacological and pharmacological treatments and to support for other coexisting conditions that may be contributing to the anxiety. Initially, the cause of the anxiety should be investigated, and appropriate non-pharmacological management given. In mild to moderate cases, psychoeducation and cognitive behavioural therapy is the first-line treatment. If the young person also has autism spectrum disorder (ASD), practical steps specifically to support ASD (e.g. implementing or re-implementing visual timetables in school) may significantly reduce anxiety. Progress should be monitored regularly, and medication should be considered in cases that are moderate to severe and/or that do not respond to or make little progress with therapy.

In a 4-month randomised controlled trial of methylphenidate for ADHD in children with and without anxiety, the presence of anxiety did not influence the response to the medication or the numbers of adverse events (Diamond et al. 1999).

A 12-week trial of atomoxetine in the treatment of ADHD and comorbid anxiety in 8- to 17-year-olds demonstrated a reduction in symptoms of both ADHD and anxiety. The only significant side effect reported was that atomoxetine treatment was associated with significantly more reports of decreased appetite and weight loss than placebo (Geller et al. 2007).

If anxiety is the cause of major impairment, or anxiety symptoms do not recede as ADHD becomes controlled, the use of medication such as selective serotonin reuptake inhibitors (SSRIs) should also be considered. Both treatments can be used together, although clinicians must be aware of possible interactions such as between atomoxetine and other medications metabolised by the cytochrome P450 pathway.

Overall, it is considered that pharmacotherapy for ADHD with either stimulants or non-stimulants should be used, and the outcomes monitored in terms of ADHD and anxiety symptoms. Treating ADHD symptoms may reduce anxiety. If it does not, then further non-pharmacological treatment or pharmacological treatment for the anxiety should be instituted alongside ADHD medication.

Depression

Evidence that demonstrates the link between depression in children and young people with ADHD and low self-esteem and peer and family difficulties suggests that there may be an opportunity to reduce the risk of later depression by earlier recognition and treatment of ADHD symptoms and by the provision of interventions that target inter-personal competence and improve self esteem and quality of life in young children with ADHD (Humphreys et al. 2013).

When a child or young person with ADHD presents with symptoms of depression, it is important, initially, to assess the severity of depression and the impact of negative experiences due to the individual's ADHD. Severe depression, particularly when associated with suicidal ideation or attempts, should be treated as a priority and seen urgently by specialist CAMHS, and multimodal support should be put in place. In general, however, both the depression and the ADHD should be treated.

In mild to moderate cases, non-pharmacological management of comorbid depression should always be considered first. This could include cognitive behavioural therapy, interpersonal therapy, non-directive supportive therapy or, in mild cases, guided self-help.

In cases where the depression is moderate to severe, unresponsive to therapy alone or associated with psychosis, medication should be considered. SSRIs of choice are fluoxetine, sertraline or citalopram. In resistant cases or those with associated psychotic symptoms, augmentation with an antipsychotic is recommended (NICE Quality Standard 48, https://www.nice.org.uk/guidance/qs48).

When pharmacological treatment is required, one medication should be introduced at a time, with the most severe and impairing difficulty being treated first and then, if impairing symptoms from the second disorder continue, treatment for this should be added. A stimulant medication will usually be the first choice to control ADHD symptoms in children and young people with comorbid major depressive disorder, but atomoxetine may be used if stimulants are contraindicated (Pliszka et al. 2006).

The relative contribution of any currently prescribed medication to the onset of depression should be reviewed. There is some evidence linking both stimulant medication and atomoxetine to a small increase in the risk of depression and suicidal ideation, so the time of onset of depression should be taken into account. In some cases, stopping the ADHD medication may be considered. Whether or not this step is taken, extremely careful ongoing monitoring is required. Recurrence of ADHD symptoms if an effective medication is withdrawn could worsen depression. Where depression is identified in an adolescent with ADHD, the potential contribution of illicit drugs to the onset of the depression should also be considered (see Chapter 15).

Sleep disorders

The first step in managing sleep disorders is to take a detailed history with a sleep diary. This should include bedtime routine, details of the sleep environment, difficulties settling, wakenings in the night and waking in the morning. The next step is to institute general sleep hygiene measures. Carers often feel they have tried to establish a good bedtime routine and feel pessimistic about success, but structured use of sleep hygiene and behavioural techniques can resolve sleep issues for perhaps 30% of those with poor sleep and provide improvement for most. The MENDS trial by Gringras et al. (2012) investigated the use of melatonin in children with neurodevelopmental difficulties and sleep problems, and used a booklet for parents on sleep entitled 'Encouraging Good Sleep Habits in Children with Learning Disabilities'. This is available to download at researchautism.net and may be useful for families with a child with ADHD.

Leading up to bedtime, an established routine gives the child clues that bedtime is coming. Exercising to the point of breathlessness at around 4 p.m. and then tea followed by perhaps bath and quiet play with the parent, increases sleep readiness. The bedroom, and in particular being in bed, should be associated with sleep not play. Colours should be calming and clutter kept to a minimum. Blackout blinds may be helpful. If a child needs light to settle, try an orange or pink light. Extinction techniques, such as leaving the child completely alone following the completion of their bedtime routine, are sometimes recommended but may not be advisable for some children and young people with ADHD as they can be cause damage to themselves or the bedroom if left alone and unsupervised.

Blue light (e.g. television or computer screens) has been shown to switch off natural (or indeed exogenous) melatonin and should be avoided before bed. This can be a real challenge for some families with entrenched problems when the child or young person is used to watching television or playing on the computer in bed. If the screens really cannot be removed, the use of orange glasses (which can be bought online) may be helpful.

Setting a consistent bedtime and wakening time is vital, but it does need to fit with that child's sleep patterns. Not all children need the same amount of sleep.

It will help to explain to parents that things are likely to get worse when changes are made and the child or young person tries to keep the status quo, before they get better. Otherwise, understandably, families often give up. Frequent supportive contact from a team member, perhaps by telephone, can be really helpful to motivate and maintain progress.

Always consider possible additional causes of sleep problems. Ask if the child snores or gasps, appears to stop breathing and sweats profusely at night. This could indicate sleep apnoea. Examine the tonsils and consider referral for a sleep study. If sleep apnoea is diagnosed, surgery may resolve the problem. Ask about discomfort in the legs or creeping, restless feelings. This may indicate restless legs syndrome (RLS). If RLS is a possibility, measure ferritin levels and, if this is less than 30ng/ml, treat with iron. A trial of clonidine or gabapentin may also be useful in RLS.

ADHD medications and sleep

Stimulant medications may cause sleep difficulties. If this possible side effect occurs, first check the timing of doses. Generally, long-acting preparations should only be given in the morning and immediate-release preparations not after teatime. Sometimes, however, if a child/young person has severe ADHD symptoms in the evening, a teatime dose of an immediate-release preparation may help provide a calmer evening and easier settling. For some children the side effect is intolerable and another medication (e.g. atomoxetine or guanfacine) may be considered. Some clinicians may add an evening dose of clonidine.

Melatonin

Some families find treating sleep onset difficulties with melatonin very helpful. Melatonin is a naturally occurring hormone produced by the pineal gland in the brain. It is involved in coordinating the body's sleep–wake cycle. The multicentre MENDS study (Gringras et al. 2012) investigated the use of melatonin to improve sleep problems in children with neurodevelopmental difficulties (not ADHD). Participants whose sleep did not improve with sleep hygiene measures were then randomly allocated to receive melatonin (between 0.5mg and 12mg depending on response) 45 minutes before bedtime, or placebo. Melatonin increased total sleep time on average by around 22 minutes. Melatonin reduced sleep onset latency measured by actigraphy by a mean of 45 minutes and was most effective for children with the longest sleep latency. Melatonin was, however, associated with earlier waking times than placebo. Adverse events were mild and similar between the two groups. Screen use will counteract melatonin and must be avoided. In clinical practice, many parents report very positive response to 2–10mg of melatonin around 45 minutes before sleep time. However, if melatonin is successful in improving sleep, a planned trial off medication should be arranged in 3–6 months to establish whether it is still needed.

For a review of sleep in children and adolescents with ADHD see Owens (2009).

Intellectual disability/general learning disability

Once a diagnosis of ADHD has been confirmed in a child or young person with learning disability, management should follow the usual pathways. Behavioural management needs to take into account the developmental level of the individual and should be started during the assessment phase. Thinking with the family about the child's developmental level can itself be very helpful to set realistic goals for behaviour.

If medication is needed it is important to remember that cardiovascular anomalies are more frequent in this group. Most cardiac problems do not mean medication cannot be used, but discussion with a paediatric cardiologist may be needed and careful monitoring is advised (see Chapter 9).

The efficacy of stimulant medication can be similar to that in other children and young people (Simonoff et al. 2013), and in this group the benefits of improvement such as increased independence and ability to handle money can be extremely positive.

Language disorders

If a language disorder is suspected, assessment and ongoing therapy will usually be via speech and language therapy. Some ADHD teams will have direct access to speech and language therapy, but, if not, knowledge of where to refer is needed.

Autism spectrum disorder

Assessment for possible ASD in individuals with ADHD should follow the usual multi-disciplinary format with input from families and school, and joint assessment with medical staff, psychology and speech and language therapy (NICE 2011).

NICE have also produced guidance on the management of ASD in children and young people (NICE 2013). This guidance recommends the use of specific social–communication interventions for the core features of autism in children and young people. These should include play-based strategies adjusted for the child's developmental level to increase joint attention, engagement and reciprocal communication. Parents, teachers and peers should be supported in understanding the individual's communication strategies and developing new methods of increasing communication.

When considering treatment strategies to support children with ADHD and ASD there are many common features (Box 11.1) and indeed management strategies for school-age children with ASD include measures that can be helpful for all those with ADHD and indeed all children at school and at home (Box 11.2).

Visual timetables help understanding by avoiding complex language and giving clarity to what is going to happen. The Interdisciplinary Community Autism Network (ICAN) produces a simple factsheet that helps families develop visual timetables for their children (http://www.ican.org.uk/~/media/Ican2/What%20We%20Do/Enquiry%20Service/Visual%20timelines%20fact%20sheet%20parents.ashx). Structure and clear routine helps to make children less anxious and to remember what is expected of them in different situations. Low-stimulation areas reduce hypersensory difficulties and minimise distraction. Social stories help children and young people to learn what is expected in

---

Box 11.1: Factors to consider in the management of children and young people with ADHD and autism spectrum disorder (ASD)

ADHD	ASD
✓ Psychoeducation	✓ Psychoeducation
✓ Education modification	✓ Education modification
✓ Behaviour therapy	✓ Behaviour therapy
✓ ? Medication	✓ ? Medication
✓ Treating coexisting difficulties	✓ Treating coexisting difficulties
✓ Supporting families	✓ Supporting families
✓ Cross agency working	✓ Cross agency working

> **Box 11.2:** Management strategies for children with autism spectrum disorder in school
>
> **Includes:**
>
> ✓ Visual timetables, structure/routine:
>
>   Supporting understanding and language development and giving clarity to what will happen and what is expected
>
> ✓ Simple concrete language:
>
>   Used when you have the child's attention to reduce misunderstanding
>
> ✓ Low stimulation areas:
>
>   Reducing sensory difficulties
>
> ✓ Social stories:
>
>   Helping the understanding of social interaction in school and beyond
>
> All of these would also be helpful for children with ADHD.

particular scenarios and to improve understanding of other people's points of view. In the UK, the National Autistic Society website describes how to write social stories to meet the needs of specific children (http://www.autism.org.uk/about/strategies/social-stories-comic-strips/how-to-write.aspx).

Clinical experience suggests that some children and young people with ASD and ADHD do not tolerate stimulant medication as well as those without ASD. However, a retrospective and prospective trial of stimulant use in children with ADHD with or without ASD found that both groups showed statistically significant improvements in the target symptoms of 'hyperactivity', 'impulsivity', 'inattention', 'oppositionality', 'aggression' and 'intermittent explosive rage'. The Clinical Global Impression-Improvement (CGI-I) also improved in each group. There was no statistically significant difference in the degree of improvement between groups, and neither tics nor repetitive behaviours worsened. Fewer side effects were actually reported in the group with ASD (Santosh et al. 2006).

Atomoxetine has also been shown to have a positive effect in an 8-week randomised controlled trial (Harfterkamp et al. 2012) and in a longer-term open label follow-up study (Harfterkamp et al. 2013). Extended-release guanfacine, a selective alpha-2 agonist, offers an additional choice (Scahill et al. 2015). In general, 'start low and go slow' seems particularly relevant in this group.

If ASD and comorbid ADHD are combined with severe behaviour difficulties that challenge those caring for them, detailed analysis is needed. Every behaviour has a message, and understanding what the child/young person is trying to communicate and the benefit the behaviour has for them underlies a successful behaviour management plan. For example, self-harming or aggressive behaviour may be prompted by anxiety, in which case management of the cause of anxiety is needed. In some cases, if there is no improvement following careful assessment of the behaviour and the use of specific behavioural management, antipsychotic medication (e.g. aripiprazole or risperidone) may be helpful. Careful monitoring with baseline and follow-up blood investigations and ECG is needed. Excessive weight gain is frequently a concern, and premedication and follow-up dietary advice around healthy eating can be a very useful preventative strategy.

Further helpful advice and resources can be found at autism.org.

Specific learning difficulties

Management of specific literacy and numeracy difficulties will usually be undertaken within schools, but some families will also access other specific services and practice interventions at home. The role of the ADHD service is to ensure the diagnosis is considered and to be able to direct families to the appropriate local services for assessment and management.

Developmental coordination disorder

There is some evidence that the use of medication to improve the core symptoms of ADHD does improve symptoms of developmental coordination disorder (DCD) and health-related quality of life in individuals with ADHD and DCD (Flapper et al. 2006, 2008). However, at least half of children with combined motor problems and ADHD will benefit from additional motor therapy. Group or individual work is helpful, and it is often particularly effective when target orientated to specific skills the child/young person wishes to master (e.g. riding a bike).

Occupational therapists and physiotherapists will provide therapy for the child/young person and input to schools so that support can continue in physical education classes.

Some simple advice to families can also be very useful (e.g. ensuring school clothes are easy to get on and off). Help packing the rucksack and lunchbox for school may be needed for longer than parents expect. Many strategies to reduce impairment caused by DCD at home, in school and during play and leisure activities can be found at www.boxofideas.org.

Motor coordination difficulties should show some ongoing improvement, although increased demand and expectation may mask this. If a deterioration of skills appears to be taking place, careful neurological examination and review of the diagnosis is essential.

Tic disorders and Tourette syndrome

If a child or young person with ADHD has tics, record the frequency and form of any tics before commencing medication. Either use a formal scale (e.g. the Yale Global Tic Severity Scale (YGTSS), available at http://dcf.psychiatry.ufl.edu/files/2011/06/TIC-YGTSS-Clinician.pdf), or simply ask the family to record tic type and frequency in a diary. Tics naturally come and go, and the frequency waxes and wanes over days or months. In the short term, boredom, anxiety and pressure to cease can increase frequency. There is still some concern that methylphenidate may increase tic frequency. However, the consensus view is that stimulants are not contraindicated in the management of ADHD in individuals who also have tics. Tic frequency should be monitored, but it is important to resist stopping successful treatment if tics increase as this may be a normal periodic increase that will soon improve. If tic frequency remains an issue or if the family express a preference, atomoxetine is a useful alternative and may actually decrease tics.

Scahill et al. (2001) investigated the use of extended-release guanfacine in a short placebo-controlled trial in a group of 31 children with combined-type ADHD and a tic disorder. After 8 weeks of treatment, guanfacine was associated with a mean improvement of 37% in the total score on the teacher-rated ADHD Rating Scale, compared to 8% improvement for placebo. Tic severity decreased by 31% in the guanfacine group, compared to 0% in the placebo group.

If tics distress the child/young person they merit treatment in their own right. Clonidine, an alpha-2 agonist, is a helpful choice and may also help with sleep and ADHD symptoms. Atypical antipsychotics can be considered if symptoms remain distressing despite behavioural and other pharmacological agents.

For a useful review of Tourette syndrome see Robertson (2012).

Epilepsy

No double-blind, placebo-controlled studies have been reported that address the efficacy of medications for ADHD in this population. However, the available open-label and preclinical trials suggest that both methylphenidate (Santos et al. 2013) and atomoxetine may be safe and efficacious (Parisi et al. 2010) and the evidence of any seizure-promoting effect is poor.

The impact of ADHD medication on seizure frequency should be closely monitored using seizure diaries, especially in the initial medication trial period. It is wise to check any possible drug interactions between ADHD medications and antiepilepsy medications. For example, if considering the use of guanfacine HCl to treat ADHD in a child with epilepsy, remember that exposure to this medication is affected by concomitant use of CYP3A4/5 inducers or inhibitors. Carbamazepine is a strong CYP3A4 inducer. If guanfacine is combined with a strong enzyme inducer, a re-titration to increase the dose up to a maximum daily dose of 7mg may be considered if needed. If the inducing treatment is ended, re-titration to reduce the guanfacine dose is recommended during the following weeks.

ADHD is currently under-diagnosed in children and young people with epilepsy. Treatment can be extremely positive for the children and their families, so an increase in recognition is needed (Shalev 2013).

Summary

- Comorbid difficulties are the rule rather than the exception, and taking them into account when assessing and managing children and young people with ADHD is essential.

- Teams will have expertise in managing some or all of the difficulties, but, otherwise, detailed knowledge of other local services and good communication and team working is required.

References

Biederman J, Spencer TJ, Newcorn JH et al. (2007) Effect of comorbid symptoms of oppositional defiant disorder on responses to atomoxetine in children with ADHD: A meta-analysis of controlled clinical trial data. *Psychopharmacology (Berl)* 190(1): 31–41.

Diamond IR, Tannock R, Schachar RJ (1999) Response to methylphenidate in children with ADHD and comorbid anxiety. *J Am Acad Child Adolesc Psychiatry* 38(4): 402–409, doi:10.1097/00004583-199904000-00012A.

Flapper BC, Houwen S, Schoemaker MM (2006) Fine motor skills and effects of methylphenidate in children with attention-deficit-hyperactivity disorder and developmental coordination disorder. *Dev Med Child Neurol* 48(3): 165–169.

Flapper BC, Schoemaker MM (2008) Effects of methylphenidate on quality of life in children with both developmental coordination disorder and ADHD. *Dev Med Child Neurol* 50(4): 294–299, doi:10.1111/j.1469-8749.2008.02039.x.

Geller D, Donnelly C, Lopez F et al. (2007) Atomoxetine treatment for pediatric patients with attention-deficit/hyperactivity disorder with comorbid anxiety disorder. *J Am Acad Child Adolesc Psychiatry* 46(9): 1119–1127, doi:10.1097/chi.0b013e3180ca8385.

Gringras P, Gamble C, Jones AP et al. and the MENDS Study Group (2012) Melatonin for sleep problems in children with neurodevelopmental disorders: Randomised double masked placebo controlled trial. *Br Med J* 345: e6664, doi:10.1136/bmj.e6664.

Harfterkamp M1Harfterkamp MI, van de Loo-Neus G, Minderaa RB et al. (2012) A randomized double-blind study of atomoxetine versus placebo for attention-deficit/hyperactivity disorder symptoms in children with autism spectrum disorder. *J Am Acad Child Adolesc Psychiatry* 51(7): 733–741, doi:10.1016/j.jaac.2012.04.011.

Harfterkamp MI, Buitelaar JK, Minderaa RB, van de Loo-Neus G, van der Gaag RJ, Hoekstra PJ (2013) Long-term treatment with atomoxetine for attention-deficit/hyperactivity disorder symptoms in children and adolescents with autism spectrum disorder: An open-label extension study. *J Child Adolesc Psychopharmacol* 23(3): 194–199, doi:10.1089/cap.2012.0012.

Humphreys KL, Katz SJ, Lee SS, Hammen C, Brennan PA, Najman JM (2013) The association of ADHD and depression: Mediation by peer problems and parent–child difficulties in two complementary samples. *J Abnorm Psychol* 122(3): 854–867, doi:10.1037/a0033895.

Jensen PS, Hinshaw SP, Kraemer HC et al. (2001) ADHD comorbidity findings from the MTA study: Comparing comorbid subgroups. *J Am Acad Child Adolesc Psychiatry* 40(2): 147–158.

Newcorn JH, Spencer TJ, Biederman J, Milton DR, Michelson D (2005) Atomoxetine treatment in children and adolescents with attention-deficit/hyperactivity disorder and comorbid oppositional defiant disorder. *J Am Acad Child Adolesc Psychiatry* 44: 240–248.

NICE (2011) *Autism diagnosis in children and young people: Recognition, referral and diagnosis of children and young people on the autism spectrum*, NICE guidelines [CG128], https://www.nice.org.uk/guidance/cg128/chapter/1-Guidance.

NICE (2013) *Autism: The management and support of children and young people on the autism spectrum*, NICE guidelines [CG170], https://www.nice.org.uk/guidance/CG170/chapter/introduction.

Owens JA (2009) A clinical overview of sleep and attention-deficit/hyperactivity disorder in children and adolescents. *J Can Acad Child Adolesc Psychiatry* 18(2): 92–102.

Parisi P, Moavero R, Verrotti A, Curatolo P (2010) Attention deficit hyperactivity disorder in children with epilepsy. *Brain Devel* 32: 10–16.

Pliszka S, Crismon ML, Carroll W et al. and the Texas Consensus Conference Panel on Pharmacotherapy of Childhood Attention-Deficit/Hyperactivity Disorder (2006) The Texas Children's Medication Algorithm Project: Revision of the algorithm for pharmacotherapy of attention-deficit/hyperactivity disorder. *J Am Acad Child Adolesc Psychiatry* 45: 642–657, doi:10.1097/01.chi.0000215326.51175.eb.

Robertson MM (2012) The Gilles De La Tourette syndrome: The current status. *Arch Dis Child Educ Pract Educ* 97: 166–175, doi:10.1136/archdischild-2011-300585.

Santos K, Palmini A, Radziuk AL et al. (2013) The impact of methylphenidate on seizure frequency and severity in children with attention-deficit-hyperactivity disorder and difficult-to-treat epilepsies. *Dev Med Child Neurol* 55(7): 654–660, doi:10.1111/dmcn.12121.

Santosh PJ, Baird G, Pityaratstian N, Tavare E, Gringras P (2006) Impact of comorbid autism spectrum disorders on stimulant response in children with attention deficit hyperactivity disorder: A retrospective and prospective effectiveness study. *Child Care Health Dev* 32(5): 575–583, doi:10.1111/j.1365-2214.2006.00631.

Scahill L, McCracken JT, King BH et al. (2015) Extended-release guanfacine for hyperactivity in children with autism spectrum disorder. *Am J Psychiatry Dec* 172(12): 1197–1206.

Scahill L, Chappell P, Kim Y et al. (2001) A placebo-controlled study of guanfacine in the treatment of children with tic disorders and attention deficit hyperactivity disorder. *Am J Psychiatry* 158(7): 1067–1074, doi:10.1176/appi.ajp.158.7.1067.

Setyawan J, Fridman M, Hodgkins P et al. (2015) Relationship between symptom impairment and treatment outcome in children and adolescents with attention-deficit/hyperactivity disorder: A physician perspective. *Atten Defic Hyperact Disord* 7(1): 75–87, doi:10.1007/s12402-014-0143-0.

Shalev R (2013) Good news: Methylphenidate for ADHD in epilepsy. *Devel Med Child Neurol* 55(7): 590–591, doi:10.1111/dmcn.12111.

Simonoff E, Taylor E, Baird G et al. (2013) Randomized controlled double-blind trial of optimal dose methylphenidate in children and adolescents with severe attention deficit hyperactivity disorder and intellectual disability. *J Child Psychol Psychiatry* 54(5): 527–535, doi:10.1111/j.1469-7610.2012.02569.x.

Van der Heijden KB, Smits MG, Van Someren EJ, Ridderinkhof KR, Gunning WB (2007) Effect of melatonin on sleep, behaviour and cognition in ADHD and chronic sleep onset insomnia. *J Am Acad Child Adolesc Psychiatry* 46: 233–241.

van der Stouwe T, Asscher J, Stams G, Deković M, van der Laan P (2014) The effectiveness of multisystemic therapy (MST): A meta analysis. *Clin Psychol Review* 34(6): 468–481, doi:10.1016/j.cpr.2014.06.006.

Weiss MD, Wasdell MB, Bomben MM, Rea KJ, Freeman RD (2006) Sleep hygiene and melatonin treatment for children and adolescents with ADHD and initial insomnia. *J Am Acad Child Adolesc Psychiatry* 45: 512–519.

Chapter 12

The role of the ADHD nurse specialist

Julie Warburton and Mel Seymour

Introduction

In this chapter we will discuss the possible role of an ADHD nurse specialist within a team involved in the assessment and management of ADHD in children and young people. The first ADHD nurse specialist role in the UK was established in around 1999. A number of posts have since been established and the benefit to services is now well established, but many teams in the UK and elsewhere still do not have anyone in this valuable role. Some ADHD specialist nurses are paediatric nurses by training, some have worked in health visiting or as school nurses, and others trained as child and adolescent mental health nurses. Some are nurse prescribers, having undertaken the additional training, but this is not essential.

General principles

There are a number of general principles that underpin the role of the specialist nurse. Often, families have been on a difficult journey prior to diagnosis, leading to a negative outlook and poor self-esteem both for parents and children. Families sometimes feel rejected and ostracised, which may increase family conflict and feelings of isolation.

The role of the nurse specialist should be one of non-judgmental support, understanding and approachability. The nurse specialist can provide a positive and productive contact, starting around the time of diagnosis, which will often be ongoing throughout the child's treatment, working with families to achieve optimal outcomes for the children and young people in their care.

At the point of diagnosis, parents may find they are unable to fully absorb the information provided and, due to time constraints within many clinic settings, there may be limited opportunity to rectify this. The nurse specialist is able to explore questions and concerns as well as provide information and signposting to other agencies and opportunities available. This may be the first time that families experience ADHD presented in a positive light, supported by the use of positive role models and a focus on achievements and aspirations for the future.

As a consistent clinician involved in the child's care, a specialist nurse is in the fortunate position of being able to see the child grow and develop over time. This provides an opportunity to form trusting relationships with both the child/young person and the family. Support is offered through clinic appointments and telephone contact, making the nurse specialist accessible not only to all families but also to other agencies as a trusted contact providing a holistic service.

Throughout time spent with the family, empowerment should remain paramount to the care delivered. Families and children should be encouraged to communicate with and to seek help from other agencies (e.g. education and support networks, parent groups). Families who communicate regularly and positively with other agencies are usually successful in achieving good outcomes for their child. With up-to-date knowledge and experience of both the public and voluntary sector as well as multiagency working, the nurse is able to signpost families in the direction of such support (Steer 2005).

Time can also be spent supporting families and young people to problem solve. Where small difficulties can be managed effectively through positive methods and encouragement, escalation into more serious problems can be prevented. Accessibility of the nurse specialist provides opportunity for early intervention.

Specific roles

An ADHD nurse specialist may undertake several specific roles in a team (Box 12.1).

Classroom observation
Structured observation in school has become the criterion standard for providing objective information in the diagnostic process and, although in some services school observations are performed by a range of professionals, in others they have become a key part of the nurse specialist role. The first contact a specialist nurse has with a child or young

---

Box 12.1: Role of the ADHD specialist nurse

✓ Accessible contact point for families, GPs and schools
✓ Provision of information to parents and schools
✓ Structured classroom observation
✓ Individual and group behavioural management for parents
✓ Nurse-led follow-up clinics
✓ Input to school or other multiagency meetings
✓ Group training for other health or education professionals
✓ Support during transition to adult services

---

person will often be in the school setting at the classroom observation. Following initial consultation and concerns raised around features of ADHD, the consulting clinician will request a school observation. The covert classroom observation can be an extremely useful tool in the diagnosis of ADHD, as a child/young person is seen in a situation they are used to, in the company of others of the same age (Box 12.2).

When arranging a time to observe the child in the classroom, key points should be taken into consideration. First the child should be completely unaware that they are being scrutinised so that they cannot modify their normal behaviour. Ideally, the observation should take place within a setting that will involve the need to sit and focus for a period of time, for example within a maths or literacy session. It may, however, be appropriate to see the child in more than one session in order to gain a true perspective on the child's abilities both to focus and to meet the demands of the teacher. It may also be beneficial to review the child within a social setting such as during a break time, particularly where there may be concerns around comorbidity. During these times, impulsivity and levels of activity can also be assessed as this often creates difficulties within the peer group.

To support accurate gathering of information, the observation is guided by the use of a behaviour time sampler specifically devised to look at the core features of ADHD within the classroom. This compares the index child with a control child suggested by

---

Box 12.2: School observation

✓ Timed observation of ADHD symptoms compared with control child
✓ General comparison with whole class on linear scale
✓ Free text comments on ADHD and possible coexisting conditions
✓ Discussion with teacher/SENCO about current difficulties and strengths
✓ Discussion about strategies used so far and additional suggestions to trial

---

the teacher, every 2 minutes, over a timed period, and in a linear form with the whole class over the full observation period. This enables all observations to be comparable and of equal quality and carried out over an agreed period of time. It offers guidance to the assessing clinician and can be clearly interpreted back in the clinic setting when providing feedback to parents alongside parent and teacher rating scales. Sometimes, if response to management is unclear or suboptimal, a second observation may be undertaken and the structured format provides robust comparisons.

The observation offers the opportunity to verify that the child is presenting with typical behaviours, but the school visit also allows the nurse to discuss the progress of the child, both academically and socially, and gain information around any existing interventions used to support them. This key information can be gained from the class teacher and special needs coordinator or key workers involved with the child's current provision. In addition, there is an opportunity to suggest specific strategies to the teacher that will help support this child with ADHD immediately. Any existing information from other agencies, such as Educational Psychology, Learning Support and the Autism Education team, should be collected to help further develop a picture of the child's needs or difficulties.

Time spent working within the classroom setting also allows the nurse specialist to form good working relationships with schools, in particular with special needs coordinators. This can lead to a robust, two-way system of support and communication between schools and the ADHD service.

Working with families

The first meeting with the parents/carers will usually be either within the clinic setting or at parent workshops. Both settings provide time to explore a child/young person's strengths and difficulties within a positive environment – something that parents may not have previously experienced.

Parent workshops

Following diagnosis, parents are encouraged to gain as much information around their child's strengths and difficulties as possible in order to support them fully. It is essential that they have a good understanding of the potential impact that ADHD may have upon both learning and social and emotional development. As recommended by NICE (2008), such needs can be met through the provision of a parent education and management course. Although meta-analysis has not clearly demonstrated a robust evidence base for parent management courses (Sonuga-Barke et al. 2014), they are highly valued by parents/carers and fulfil a number of needs in the support package.

The nurse specialist is well placed within a support role to provide such information for carers and to be one of the facilitators for the workshops. Although it gives an opportunity to empower parents to manage their child's difficulties both at home and within the school setting, it also creates time during which a good working relationship between parents and the service can be developed. Parents are able to meet with other parent/carers having similar experiences, often helping each other to problem-solve and gain confidence in managing their child's condition. Parents may have had negative experiences of such groups, so it is essential that the group is facilitated by an experienced practitioner who can create and maintain a positive outlook.

In order to provide a comprehensive and informative package of education around ADHD, the group should run over several weeks (NICE 2008). This enables all aspects of the condition and its management to be explored. It also provides a period of time following information and strategies being given for changes to be made and measured within a supportive and non-judgmental environment. The sessions (Box 12.3) should include advice and information regarding the condition itself and the likely effects of core features on their children. It should then focus on the management of this through strategies such as boundary setting and reward and consequence. The development of robust routines should be a key discussion area, as well the use of tools such as visual aids to support this. A full session should be dedicated to the use of medication, allowing parents time to discuss options and concerns such as effects and side effects, as well as dispel any myths they may have heard. For many this may be the first opportunity they have had to consider this in detail in a relaxed setting alongside others who may already have had experience. A clinician working with ADHD medications on a regular basis should therefore deliver this session.

The course should support parents to consider their expectations of their child in line with the child's difficulties, developmental level and cognitive ability. It should encourage them to review how they talk to their child and place demands on them in everyday life. While promoting positivity, it should provide parents with strategies to maintain this with their children as well as helping their child to grow in confidence and independence. It is also vital that parents are encouraged to consider their own well-being and support, as meeting the needs of a child with ADHD can be very demanding.

Box 12.3: The Managing ADHD course for parents and carers in Sheffield, UK

✓ **Week 1** Understanding ADHD
✓ **Week 2** Organising and structuring
✓ **Week 3** Communication
✓ **Week 4** Medication
✓ **Week 5** Behaviour
✓ **Week 6** Activities and resources
✓ **Week 7** Coping and family
✓ **Week 8** Evaluate and celebrate

Teacher training

The progress of the child is greatly affected by experiences, both academic and social, within the school setting. Teachers are in a prime position to have a direct influence on the child's self-esteem and confidence, and a child whose needs around ADHD are met within school is much more likely to achieve his or her potential. In order for teachers to provide this level of academic, social and emotional support, a good understanding of ADHD is required. As it is estimated that at least one or two children in every class of 30 will present with significant features of ADHD, training around the condition would seem appropriate for all teaching and classroom support staff, especially as many strategies used in its management will be of benefit to all children.

Ideally, teachers in training should learn about general strategies to support pupils with special needs, including those with ADHD; however, the time available to do this is limited. Also, each child with ADHD and other special needs is unique and presents with their own individual needs. The nurse specialist is in a position to offer education around support and strategies both for all children with ADHD and specific to the individual child. Training can therefore be delivered during planned group sessions or on an ad-hoc or opportunistic basis.

Support and training within the classroom often begins at the point of school observation. During this time key, concerns may be raised, for example about poor listening skills or inability to cope with sitting on the carpet. This may in turn generate suggestions around how this may be managed such as being placed at the front of a classroom or being provided with a chair at carpet time. Small changes can make a huge difference to the child's ability to cope within the classroom. Such changes may not have previously been considered due to limited knowledge of the causes of behaviours.

Where possible, teachers will benefit from being provided with the same quality of information that parents receive. Time constraints and funding can impede this, and training cannot always be offered on the same basis as parent education. Despite this, it remains beneficial to hold group sessions for school staff to provide an overview of the condition, strategies for management and support available. This should include verbal and written information in line with that given to parents. The nurse specialist contact details should be offered for use where problems or concerns arise or simply to request advice. The session should also offer the opportunity to discuss gaps in knowledge and problem-solving skills centred on ADHD, when presented with difficulties in the classroom.

Teachers should also be made aware of the beneficial effects and potential side effects of medication. Good practice within medical management of ADHD requires feedback from and effective communication with school in order to titrate and optimise treatment. A knowledge of what medication can and cannot do and realistic expectations of treatment can significantly help both the teacher and clinician to monitor the child's progress effectively.

Nurse-led clinics

The nurse specialist is ideally placed to follow up and support children diagnosed with ADHD within nurse-led clinics. Although all children continue to be seen at regular intervals by a member of the medical team or prescribing clinician, much of their support is based around the school environment and how ADHD impacts upon everyday life both there at home. With high levels of contact with both schools and parents, the nurse is in a position to offer support using a holistic and child centred approach.

Clinic appointments should be of reasonable length in order to provide time to discuss progress and problems. Many children feel comfortable enough to speak to a nurse in a relaxed environment, and appointments are kept as informal as possible to allow the child to contribute to discussion. Where possible, the consultation is directed towards the child, allowing them to become involved in their own care. It is important that the child develops an understanding of ADHD and the reasoning behind clinic appointments. The nurse can use clinic appointments as an opportunity to develop trusting relationships with the child, enhancing the links between children, parents, the medical team and school.

During all clinic appointments, some key points of discussion need to be raised. First, progress at school academically, socially and emotionally should be considered. Where concerns are raised it is then appropriate to make contact with school to follow up any concerns and gain a full picture. For children taking medication to manage symptoms, the use of a rating scale completed both by school and parents may be helpful in benchmarking its efficacy. In addition, specific goals chosen in discussion with the child/young person and family should be established and reviewed, perhaps using a visual scale or other agreed measure (e.g. numbers of detentions). In some cases, re-observation within the classroom may be necessary. With good school links this can be a straightforward task following the clinic appointment.

Equally, home life should be discussed, gaining both the child and parental perspective. For children it is often appropriate and insightful for the young person to be seen alone at the beginning of the appointment. The nurse specialist has often been a constant and familiar face within consultations, so many children feel comfortable discussing sensitive issues. The nurse may have some time to discuss issues around healthy lifestyle and risk taking relevant to the child's age and developmental levels, such as smoking, relationships or driving. It also provides the opportunity to empower children to move towards independence and more control over their own difficulties.

Specific monitoring is also essential where drug therapy is used (NICE 2008). The nurse specialist needs to have an excellent understanding of the medication used in the management of ADHD, taking into consideration the potential risks and benefits at all clinic appointments. Both growth and cardiovascular effects need to be carefully monitored at each visit. These should take into account blood pressure, pulse, height, weight (all compared with standard charts) and appetite. Alongside these, effects upon sleep are an important factor to be considered.

Because of the level of contact, the nurse specialist is well placed to titrate medication according to the impact of symptoms on the child. This should be done using a validated assessment tool such as a rating scale. Ideally, both parents and the school should provide information in order to build a full picture of the child's progress and to support the change. Any changes made should be completed within an agreed protocol, including limits of treatment, and followed up appropriately. This can be carried out over the phone or face to face.

As changes to medication are frequently made, it is important to build good relationships with general practitioners (GPs). In the majority of cases, where GPs are in agreement, they will be asked to prescribe through the guidance of a shared care protocol. Contact details should be made available to GPs so that medication concerns can be discussed and, where needed, the nurse specialist can provide information around treatment and monitoring.

Decisions regarding follow-up intervals can be made depending on the outcomes of the current appointment, but should be at least 6-monthly according to NICE guidelines (2008).

Team working
The ADHD nurse specialist is, like any other member, part of an overall team supporting the child/young person and their family. The diagnosis and management of ADHD is a team process, and regular effective communication, skill sharing and mutual respect are essential among core team members, including medical and psychology staff, as well as other professionals such as teachers, speech and language therapists and physiotherapists. Team support and mutual supervision is especially important in our working environment, which can often be stressful and complex.

Summary

- The ADHD nurse specialist is uniquely placed within the service to offer a holistic and child-centred approach to managing ADHD in line with NICE guidance, The Children Act (2004) and Every Child Matters (Treasury 2003) outcomes.

- The process of care should encourage staying safe, being healthy both mentally and physically, enjoying and achieving, making a positive contribution and achieving economic well-being.

- All these factors can be considered within the outcomes of ADHD and so can be built into each and every contact and into daily practice.

- Every child or young person with ADHD remains an individual with changing needs at each phase of their development.

- The nurse specialist is in a fortunate and unique position to offer ongoing and comprehensive support, through medical, social and emotional management up to the point of transition into adulthood. The opportunity to provide such a level of support should significantly enhance successful outcomes for the child's future.

References

NICE (2008) *Attention deficit hyperactivity disorder: Diagnosis and management.* NICE Clinical Guidelines [CG72], https://www.nice.org.uk/guidance/cg72.

Treasury (2003) *Every child matters.* London: Stationery Office, ISBN 0101586027.

Steer CR (2005) Managing attention deficit/hyperactivity disorder: Unmet needs and future directions. *Arch Dis Child* 90: i19–i25, doi:10.1136/adc.2004.059352.

Sonuga-Barke E, Brandeis D, Holtmann M, Cortese S (2014) Computer-based cognitive training for ADHD: A review of current evidence. *Child Adolesc Psychiatr Clin N Am* 23(4): 807–824, doi:10.1016/j.chc.2014.05.009.

Chapter 13

Young people and ADHD

Caroline Bleakley

Far more than half a dozen of one… and six of the other…

(Inattentive, hyperactive, impulsive – DSM-5 symptoms)

I don't want to take this any more. It makes me too sensible.

(David aged 12 years)

Case scenario: Callum

Callum is seen for review of his ADHD aged 11.

He started secondary school a few months earlier. He has been getting frequent warnings and now detentions for not having the correct equipment in lessons. He is in even more trouble for forgetting detention.

He reacts angrily at home, hitting out at his brother and at school shouting back at the teachers.

His Mum feels that his ADHD is 'worsening' and wonders if the medication he takes (extended release methylphenidate) needs increasing.

In this chapter we will work to develop an understanding of some of the specific challenges that young people growing up with ADHD have to face. There are several changes that take place for all young people as they move into adolescence. For a young person with ADHD these changes interact with their ADHD, with the risk of even greater turmoil. It is helpful to consider separately the changes in the young people themselves, changes to their ADHD, and changes they will meet in the world around them, and then consider how all these issues may interact for the individual young person (Boxes 13.1–13.3).

Box 13.1: Changes in the young person

✓ They will enter and move through the physical and hormonal changes of puberty
✓ They will want to become more independent, like their peers, exerting autonomy and moving away from their parents
✓ They will want to develop new relationships with their own and perhaps the opposite sex

BUT

✓ **They will have slower maturation of the neural networks in the brain than their peers with an emotional maturity about 3 years behind their peers**

Box 13.2: Changes in the young person's ADHD

ADHD core symptoms

✓ Persistent inattention and impulsivity
✓ Reduction of motor restlessness
✓ Difficulty in planning and organisation
✓ Difficulty starting tasks and sustaining effort

Possible associated difficulties

✓ Aggressive, antisocial and delinquent behaviour
✓ Alcohol and drug problems
✓ Social/relationship difficulties (more vulnerable to positive or negative influences)
✓ Anxiety and/or depression
✓ Accidents

Box 13.3: Changes in the environment

✓ More independence is expected at home, school, college or work
✓ Less supervision = more risk (e.g. accidents)
✓ Availability of cigarettes, alcohol/drugs, legal 'highs'
✓ Friendships and relationships more complex, including opportunity for sexual experimentation
✓ Increased exposure to social media
✓ Driving

Brain maturation in young people with ADHD

The typically developing brain goes through a well-defined process of maturation between childhood and adulthood. There is initial cortical thickening, starting at the back of the brain and moving forward to the prefrontal cortex last of all. After reaching a peak, there follows a phase of further cortical maturation associated with cortical thinning as pathways and connections are refined (apoptosis). In individuals with ADHD the cortical maturation process follows the same pattern as that of the typically developing brain but appears to be delayed by several years (on average between 2 and 5 years behind in different brain areas in a group of children at a mean age of 10 years) (Gogtay et al. 2004; Shaw et al. 2007).

The environment

There are also new challenges facing the young person in their secondary school environment (Box 13.4). These can be considered in the areas of learning, social demands and organisation. As a young person moves through secondary school they have to cope with lecture style learning, taking notes that can be referred to later, understanding homework assignments and working independently and in a team.

Social relationships with peers become more complex, requiring sophisticated navigation between defined friendship groups. Young people need to understand the banter/language of each group, how to behave in different situations, and how to mingle appropriately with the opposite sex. It is necessary to adapt to many different teaching styles (e.g. which teacher is being sarcastic, who is telling a joke and who is absolutely

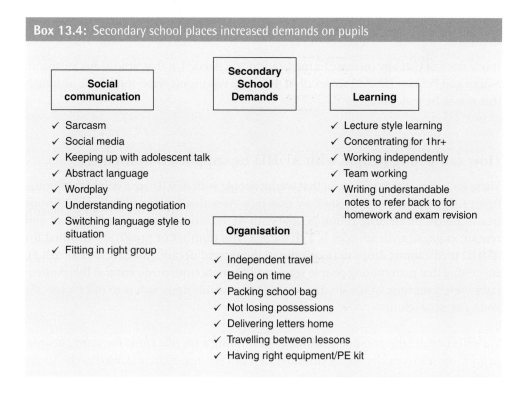

Box 13.4: Secondary school places increased demands on pupils

Secondary School Demands

Social communication
- ✓ Sarcasm
- ✓ Social media
- ✓ Keeping up with adolescent talk
- ✓ Abstract language
- ✓ Wordplay
- ✓ Understanding negotiation
- ✓ Switching language style to situation
- ✓ Fitting in right group

Learning
- ✓ Lecture style learning
- ✓ Concentrating for 1hr+
- ✓ Working independently
- ✓ Team working
- ✓ Writing understandable notes to refer back to for homework and exam revision

Organisation
- ✓ Independent travel
- ✓ Being on time
- ✓ Packing school bag
- ✓ Not losing possessions
- ✓ Delivering letters home
- ✓ Travelling between lessons
- ✓ Having right equipment/PE kit

serious). A high degree of organisation and personal responsibility is expected, such as being able to move around a large number of classrooms and school sites and arriving on time with the right equipment.

Let us think about one young person's experience. Callum was introduced at the beginning of the chapter. Although Callum is 11 years old, he is likely to be functioning emotionally more in line with an 8-year-old, and yet he is being expected to walk independently to school for the first time, cross busy roads, pack his own school bag, move between and find his way around five lessons each day, bring the right equipment, concentrate through 5 hours of lecture style learning, bring homework in on time, and much more.

Callum has been coming to the clinic for two and a half years and knows the team well. He says he is really fed up and feels angry and down. In this case, our ADHD nurse was able to attend a school meeting, which included Callum, to discuss ways of supporting Callum and ensure that all of his 11 new teachers were aware of his ADHD diagnosis. His mum decided she would support him to pack his bag each evening to give him a good start the next day. She also decided she would drop him off at school for a while longer as she was uncertain about his road safety when crossing busier roads. Teachers agreed to remind him to give in pieces of work (often previously done but left in his bag) and to e-mail any lesson presentations home along with homework instructions. With support in place, Callum felt more able to manage the new challenges in school and he was less angry at home and school.

It was not felt that any increase to medication was needed at that time as his Swanson, Nolan and Pelham (SNAP) scores of ADHD core symptoms were optimized, although this was to be reviewed.

How can young people with ADHD be supported optimally?

There is clear evidence to suggest that young people with ADHD are a vulnerable group. Box 13.5 gives some of the risks they may face. As with all young people with chronic health needs, motivating young people with ADHD to continue with treatment and remain engaged with services is a challenge. The number of prescriptions filled for ADHD medications drops dramatically in the second decade (McCarthy et al. 2012), suggesting that many young people who would benefit from medication at this particularly important time of life do not use it. One possible approach is to offer a specific young persons' clinic.

We will consider the possible advantages of running a specific clinic for young people, helpful topics to consider during clinical review of a young person, and also the challenges in preparing for transition into adult services.

> **Box 13.5:** What does research tell us about what might happen for young persons with ADHD?
>
> When compared with young people who do not have ADHD they are:
>
> ✓ Three times more likely be involved in an accident as the driver and more likely to be injured or injure others
> ✓ Seven times more likely to have had at least two significant accidents by adulthood
> ✓ Sexually active at a younger age
> ✓ Four times more likely to catch sexually transmitted diseases
> ✓ Ten times more likely to give birth at less than 20 years of age
>
> (Barkley 2004; Barkley et al. 2010)
>
> ✓ More likely to have been arrested and convicted
>
> (Mannuzza et al. 2008; Harpin & Young 2012)
>
> Substances
>
> ✓ More likely to smoke at age less than 15
> ✓ Two to three times more likely to abuse tobacco
> ✓ Three to eight times more likely to abuse alcohol
> ✓ Eight times more likely to develop drug dependence and to remain addicted for longer
>
> (Wilens 2007; see Chapter 16)

What do young people think about their ADHD?

The move to secondary school is a really useful time to explore what young people understand about their ADHD. Many have been coming to clinic since early primary years but, despite their best efforts, clinicians may not have had ample opportunity to talk at length with the children themselves, as consultations with younger children can often be parent-led, focusing mainly on the agenda and concerns of the parent/carers. Young people may be left with a very negative understanding of what ADHD is, possibly due to media interpretation, and generally reflecting others' negative views of them.

One of the first 'jobs' when a young person comes to the clinic is to talk to them directly and usually alone, to fully explore their current understanding of ADHD. Box 13.6 lists responses from young people joining the young persons' clinic in Sheffield who were asked 'What is ADHD?' While acknowledging their concerns, this is also an opportunity to recognise and stress a young person's strengths, and help them to see and value them.

The Voices project led by Illina Singh (http://www.adhdvoices.com) gives a clear insight into young people's views of their ADHD and ADHD medications. It is important to take on board the positive feedback young people gave about contact with their clinicians and about the overall effects of medication.

> **Box 13.6:** What do young people understand about their ADHD?
>
> ADHD is:
>
> ✓ Bad behaviour
> ✓ Why I can't control myself
> ✓ Anger issues
> ✓ Why people don't like me
> ✓ Abuse disorder
> ✓ It's my bad temper and anger
> ✓ When I get giddy and when I get sent out of class
> ✓ Concentration and poor reading
>
> (Young people's views in Sheffield service Jan/Feb 2014)

Let us consider another young person's views and needs and possible responses. Cameron, who is 14 years old, came to clinic for review with both his parents. He appeared very low. Time was spent with Cameron on his own, exploring his understanding of ADHD and how it affected him. To Cameron, ADHD meant 'getting sent out of class', 'bad behaviour' and 'getting into trouble' at school and then at home. Everything felt very negative to him. Further discussion, however, revealed strengths in a strong interest in building very creative model go-karts, great energy and stamina. How ADHD was affecting him, and why, was explored using pictures and descriptions of the brain chemistry. Medication was explained in more detail and with emphasis on what can and cannot be achieved. At this point, Cameron disclosed that he was often not swallowing his medication, even though his parents gave it to him and thought that he was. Parent and teacher SNAP scores reflecting ADHD core symptoms confirmed that his control was still suboptimal on days when he did take the medication and very poor on days when he did not. Cameron decided to increase his medication, take it regularly and join in a telephone review 2 weeks later. Boxes 13.7 and 13.8 review Cameron's case.

Seeing the young person alone helps them to become used to talking for themselves before moving into adult settings, makes it more likely that they will give honest answers, gives essential information about social communication and other comorbidity, helps to build a relationship with the clinician, and most importantly gives the best chance of their views or any specific concerns they may have being heard. Sometimes, the benefits are clearly seen by a complete transformation, with change in posture from quiet and hunched when parents do all of the talking to opening up as their views become a clear and valued part of the picture.

Using examples of popular, famous people with ADHD can also be helpful.

Box 13.7: What does ADHD mean to Cameron?

His perceptions

- ✓ 'Getting sent out of class'
- ✓ 'Bad behaviour'
- ✓ 'Getting into trouble' at school and then at home

Current specific issues

- ✓ Butts in queues
- ✓ Calls out
- ✓ Drives go-kart recklessly

His current worries

- ✓ Will he get the grades to go on into sixth form?
- ✓ If not, what happens next?
- ✓ Feels down and anxious

ADHD control

- ✓ SNAP score: 32 (parents)
  40 (school)
- ✓ Admits to often forgetting medication

Box 13.8: Focus in clinic on this occasion

Consider positives and how to build on them

- ✓ Talented builder of model go-karts. Discuss sharing this skill and safe driving of the finished go-karts
- ✓ Celebrate high energy and stamina
- ✓ Agree achievable goals

Formulate plan together

- ✓ Discuss ADHD and how medication can help
- ✓ Trial increase of long-acting stimulant with telephone review in 2 weeks
- ✓ Share his concerns with parents and school
- ✓ Look at careers guidance and options in sixth form and in colleges and employment

Focusing on what the young person can do and what they want to achieve, while setting goals for the challenges posed by their situations and their ADHD, helps to problem-solve and promote independence. The young person bringing their own ideas into the discussion and decision-making increases their motivation and engagement.

Communicating with young people

Effective communication is key to maintaining engagement when working with young people. Bombarding a young person with questions is likely to lead to confusion and no or minimal response. Time to process questions is needed to elicit true information and facilitate discussion.

In the face of a crisis consultation, the power of a warm human interaction and reception from a familiar clinician with the ability to listen should not be underestimated. Positive upbeat language, with non-judgmental comments and enquiries, is essential. 'I've heard things have been difficult recently. Tell me more' is more likely to elicit a constructive response than 'Your violent behaviour is a massive problem.' This, of course, does not mean condoning misdemeanours, but means calmly listening to the young person's thoughts as to how and why they happened. This approach will be more likely to encourage openness and to support working together to prevent further incidents. It is also important, however, to set limits and boundaries and not allow ADHD to become an excuse for more harmful behaviours.

Parent/carer involvement

It is still vital to speak to parents/carers at each appointment and to find time to have some of the consultation together. Long-term follow-up data (Barkley et al. 2002) demonstrate that young people with ADHD may be in their late twenties before they can accurately report their own symptoms and appreciate the effect they have on others. Indeed, even after transition to adult services, involvement of parents or partners can be key to maintaining engagement.

Information from other sources

Gathering information from other sources who interact with the individual with ADHD remains important too. Teachers or work colleagues may be helpful, although the young person's consent to request information is essential. Such information should then provide important topics for discussion and areas to include in management plans.

Lifestyle information and advice

It is important to focus specific discussion around the challenges today's young people are likely to meet. All of the difficult areas any young person has to navigate while growing up are magnified for young people with neurodevelopmental and mental health needs. Meeting with young people in clinic settings to review the management of their ADHD provides a useful opportunity to try to preempt difficulties or recognise them as early as possible and offer support. A familiar adult who is seen as interested can ask about lifestyle, hopefully receive honest answers, discuss options and provide resources for the young person to gain relevant information and move towards informed choices.

It is important to be honest from the outset and be clear that although the majority of discussions can remain confidential, issues that raise safeguarding concerns must be shared.

Ongoing education or employment

Every consultation should include discussion around education and or employment. Focus on what has gone well initially and then ask if there are areas for improvement, or any goals to pursue. Ask about any dreams or aspirations for the future, but give an assurance that many adolescents do not have specific ideas about their future or careers. Young people can be guided to beneficial links with education and other agencies who can then investigate with the young person the options available for further education, apprenticeships or employment.

It is important to stress that ADHD should not be seen inappropriately as a barrier to positive aspirations for the future and to try to keep realistic options open.

Hobbies and interests

Studies confirm what common sense tells us: adolescents who are kept busy in extra-curricular activities and interests are less likely to get themselves into trouble (Guindon 2009). Encouraging appropriate leisure activities, especially where positive friendships can be developed, is beneficial.

For those already making wrong choices, community youth teams may be able to direct them into activities or clubs and help the young person recognise areas of strength and ways to make positive friendships.

Smoking, alcohol and substance use

Cigarettes, alcohol and recreational drugs are often readily available to young people. Those with ADHD are by nature impulsive risk takers, and evidence shows that they are at increased risk of trying substances at a younger age, moving on quickly to even more harmful substances and developing addiction (Wilens 2007). Chapter 15 considers substance misuse in more detail. Many young people do not consider cannabis a drug, so it is helpful to ask about this separately. Legal highs are also easily available and, although perceived as safer by young people, these can be even more dangerous. Motivational interviewing (McCambridge & Strang 2004) has been shown to be effective in supporting young people to make healthier lifestyle choices. Even one meeting looking at the pros and cons of taking substances in a non-judgmental way, making a simple written list of pros and cons on opposite sides of a piece of paper, can result in a young person rethinking their decisions. If an established problem comes to light, young people should be referred to specific support services such as a community youth team or substance misuse services.

Friendships and relationships

It is important to talk to young people about their friends to find out about their support networks and also uncover any possibly negative influences. Young people with ADHD find peer relationships difficult to understand as language and inference become more complex and more abstract. Girls who had friendships in primary school may now struggle. Their immature social and emotional development often means they are more likely to be accepted by boys. Often, 'signals' may be misinterpreted, and morale-boosting attention can rapidly turn into flirtatious behaviour and lead to inappropriate sexual activity. Early sexual activity is also seen in young men with ADHD.

Reviews offer an opportunity to discuss relationships: Have they got a girlfriend/ boyfriend? Are they sexually active and what steps will they take to keep themselves and their partners safe and avoid unwanted pregnancy?

Social media

Social media merits a particular mention. There has been a great deal of change over recent times, and social media now plays a huge role in the lives of children and young people. Although this can be hugely positive for some young people with social communication difficulties, who find face-to-face contact a challenge, it is an area full of possible danger for the young person with ADHD who is impulsive and lacks social understanding. Postings easily cascade to a wider audience than intended without a teenager leaving their bedroom and can cause major problems with peers and teachers. Asking specifically about sites they are using, if they have experienced any difficulty or any cyber bullying can raise awareness and help young people and their families resolve or avoid issues. Many schools now have specific teachers who can help and advise.

Sleep

All young people go through changes of sleep patterns as they move from childhood to adult patterns. Often they go through a period when they cannot settle well and find difficulty getting up in the morning. Young people with ADHD may already have poor sleep and this may be exacerbated further by some ADHD medications. It is useful to have a general discussion around sleep needs and sleep hygiene. The screens many young people use at bedtime emit blue light, which switches off endogenous or exogenous melatonin. Those with good sleep patterns can cope with this, but sleep onset is often delayed. Screen-based activities should be avoided in the hour before settling to sleep whenever possible. Red and orange light does not inhibit melatonin action, so if a young person refuses to stop using screens, advice around modifying the screen or using orange tinted glasses (available online) can be helpful.

Driving

It is important to have a specific discussion with young people and their parents about driving, before they are eligible to apply for a provisional licence. In the UK, having a diagnosis of ADHD is not a barrier to obtaining a provisional or full driving licence, but it should be declared or the young person's insurance may be affected in the event of an accident. Both parents and young people themselves can appreciate a factual discussion about the delayed brain maturation process in ADHD, perhaps including a visual representation. Remind them that at the age of 17 years a young person with ADHD is often emotionally around 12 years old and is unlikely to have developed the good judgment needed for roadside decisions, even though manually controlling the vehicle may not be a problem.

Phillip Anderton has developed an excellent website (www.adhdandjustice.co.uk) to which young people can be directed, and a specific driving guidance leaflet can be printed off and handed to each young person and their parent/carer. Once a full licence is obtained it is important to drive at first in daylight, and without the distraction of other young people in the vehicle. An adult should accompany the young driver, even after passing the test, until that adult feels the driver has matured and has developed the good judgment necessary for driving.

Criminal activity

Where young people have made wrong choices and are coming into contact with the criminal justice system, it is important to look at available local support agencies such as community youth teams or forensic CAMHS. The website www.adhdandjustice.co.uk has a downloadable information sheet that can be handed to police outlining ADHD-specific considerations and the rights of a young person in custody.

Having ADHD is not an excuse for criminal activity. However, having ADHD makes it even more difficult to understand the complex criminal justice system, and evidence clearly illustrates that individuals with ADHD do not cope well. They frequently make false confessions to escape the situation. The Bradley Report (2009) (Box 13.9) considers the necessary additional measures needed to support individuals with learning disabilities and mental health problems.

A review, 'The challenge of ADHD and youth offending' (Harpin & Young 2012), is well worth reading.

Comorbidity

Comorbidity may become more impairing as young people are exposed to more complex demands. For example, autism spectrum disorder (ASD) may require specific support as the social demands of secondary school increase, cognitive profiles should be requested from school for anyone struggling academically or working outside the band of average, and anxiety and mood disorders are seen increasingly frequently in this age group, particularly in girls, meaning that there should be a low threshold for assessing further.

Medication choices

Young people should be fully involved in any discussions and decisions around their medications. Many will be interested in an explanation about how medications work and what they can and cannot realistically expect them to do. Treatment goals should be agreed together and scored on a simple scale to monitor progress. Optimising using SNAP scores also helps the young person and their family to understand their progress over time, and goals that are achieved always merit celebration.

The young person, and not just the parent, should be asked about side effects, as always. Appetite suppression and slow growth are particularly upsetting as classmates undergo

---

Box 13.9: Recommendations for policing and community care from the Bradley Report Executive Summary (2009)

✓ Mental health awareness and learning disabilities should be a key component in the police training programme.

✓ All police custody suites should have access to liaison and diversion services. These services would include improved screening and identification of individuals with mental health problems or learning disabilities, providing information to police and prosecutors to facilitate the earliest possible diversion of offenders with mental disorders from the criminal justice system, and signposting to local health and social care services as appropriate.

✓ Liaison and diversion services should also provide information and advice services to all relevant staff including solicitors and appropriate adults.

growth spurts, and should be minimised by encouraging the intake of calories, for example, with nutritious meals for both supper and tea, when medications are likely to have worn off.

Compliance

There are often times when young people decide that they do not want to take medications. Sometimes they will admit to this, sometimes they will hide it. When non-compliance comes to light, it is always worth asking specifically why? Sometimes it is a simple mis-understanding or concern that can be resolved. For example, a side effect that distresses the young person (e.g. lack of appetite) should be investigated and hopefully addressed.

Sometimes parents are very concerned about ADHD symptoms, but the young person is not. Young people with ADHD are frequently poor at recognising and reporting their symptoms and do not always appreciate any positive medication effects. First, it is of course necessary to discuss the concerns the parents have and any information from school with the young person and try to reach concordance. An agreed short trial away from medication with feedback from the young person, family and from teaching staff, often using specific measures (e.g. frequency of problems in school), can be persuasive, giving the young person the control to discontinue medication and indeed stay off medication if difficulties do not arise but also the choice to restart if they are given and able to experience clearer evidence of the difficulties.

In such situations, quantitative behaviour testing can also be very helpful. This comput-erised test of activity level, attention and impulsivity takes the emphasis away from the parent or clinician telling the young person what to do and allows the young person to gather visual evidence of the presence or indeed absence of ADHD symptoms. A test can be performed off and on medication to demonstrate any effects. When this objec-tive measurement, where the young person can see their own profile compared with that of a typically developing age- and sex-matched control, shows ongoing difficulties, it can give a very powerful message and young people have often made the decision themselves to restart medication.

Transition into adult services

As we have discussed, many young people disengage from services and do not make a successful transition to adult services.

Some steps that may increase engagement have already been described:

- increasing understanding of ADHD and its possible consequences;
- looking at issues young people face;

- increased involvement of young people in treatment choices;

- building up confidence and independence.

Joint working over the transition and strong networking between children's and adult services need to be established. NICE (2008) gives helpful guidance about the services needed, and Chapter 16 discusses transfer to adult services in more detail.

Young people's clinics

Increasingly, specific clinics for young people are being set up. This allows the venue, timing, environment, staff and available resources to be tailored to young people's needs. Box 13.10 summarises the benefits of such a clinic.

Box 13.10: What are the advantages of a specific young person's clinic?

The aim is to improve adherence, provide relevant lifestyle information and to motivate young people with ADHD to remain in services.

✓ Dedicated familiar clinicians build rapport and relationships. Young people may be more likely to discuss issues honestly in presence of familiar clinician

✓ Can be held at a quieter time, afternoon/early evening when young people are more likely to attend

✓ Increased time to see teenagers alone and later with family/partners

✓ Talking to young people about their ADHD can be emphasised

✓ Clinicians (doctors and specialist nurses) are tuned into young people's issues and have additional expertise in communicating with young people

✓ Specific issues relating to treatment such as goals and compliance and choices of medication include young people

✓ Age-appropriate lifestyle advice with relevant information/leaflets at hand (e.g. smoking, drinking, driving, relationships) can be shared

✓ Further education/apprenticeship/employment can be considered

✓ Issues surrounding ADHD in teenage girls become more apparent

✓ Positive interactions with criminal justice systems can be supported

✓ Preparation for transition to adult services takes place

Summary

- Young people with ADHD have many challenges to meet and overcome if they are to successfully negotiate the years between childhood and the responsibilities of adult life.

- They need to understand their ADHD and the way it affects them and the advantages and disadvantages of treatment.

- The world around them is complex and includes a plethora of likely adverse attractions and experiences. They will need to be informed about these and be able to seek help to deal with them before becoming involved in them.

- Services for young people must work to meet these special requirements and one way to do this is to develop a specific young persons' service staffed by trained professionals held at appropriate times and in appropriate venues.

- Much can be done to help young people with ADHD navigate through adolescence and to achieve their potential as adults.

Useful links for young people

- www.adhdandjustice.co.uk (includes useful information on driving)

- http://www.youngminds.org.uk/for_children_young_people/whats_worrying_you/adhd

- https://www.nice.org.uk/guidance/cg72/ifp/chapter/information-for-young-people-with-adhd

References

Barkley RA, Fischer M, Smallish L, Fletcher K (2002) The persistence of attention-deficit/hyperactivity disorder into young adulthood as a function of reporting source and definition of disorder. *J Abnorm Psychol* 111: 279–289.

Barkley R, Murphy K, Fischer M (2010) *ADHD in adults: What the science says.* Guilford Press, New York, NY.

Barkley R (2004) Driving impairments in teens and adults with attention-deficit/hyperactivity disorder. *Psychiatr Clin North Am* 27: 233–260.

Bradley Report (2009) DH Publications, London.

Gogtay N, Giedd J, Lusk L et al. (2004) Dynamic mapping of cortical development during childhood through early adulthood. *Proc Natl Acad Sci USA* 101(21): P8174–8179.

Guindon M (ed.) (2009) *Self-esteem across the lifespan.* Routledge, Abingdon.

Harpin V, Young S (2012) The challenge of ADHD and youth offending. *CEPiP* 1: 138–143.

Mannuzza S, Klein R, Moulton J (2008) Lifetime criminality among boys with attention deficit hyperactivity disorder: A prospective follow-up study into adulthood using official arrest records. *Psychiatry Res* 160(3): 237–246.

McCambridge J, Strang J (2004) The efficacy of single-session motivational interviewing in reducing drug consumption and perceptions of drug-related risk and harm among young people: Results from a multi-site cluster randomized trial. *Addiction* 99(1): 39–52.

McCarthy S, Wilton L, Murray ML, Hodgkins P, Asherson P, Wong IC (2012) The epidemiology of pharmacologically treated attention deficit hyperactivity disorder (ADHD) in children, adolescents and adults in UK primary care. *BMC Pediatr* 12: 78.

NICE (2008) *Attention deficit hyperactivity disorder: Diagnosis and management.* NICE Clinical Guidelines [CG72], https://www.nice.org.uk/guidance/cg72.

Shaw P, Eckstrand K, Sharp W et al. (2007) ADHD is characterised by a delay in cortical maturation. *Proc Natl Acad Sci USA* 104(49): 19649–19654.

Wilens T (2007) The nature of the relationship between attention-deficit/hyperactivity disorder and substance use. *J Clin Psychiatry* 68(S11): 4–8.

Young S, Murphy C, Coghill D (2011) Avoiding the 'twilight zone': Recommendations for the transition of services from adolescence to adulthood for young people with ADHD. *BMC Psychiatry* 11: 174.

Chapter 14

Girls and young women with ADHD

Nicholas Myttas

Case scenario: Sophie

Sophie first came to clinic aged 14. She arrived with her mother who is a nurse and her father who works as an ambulance driver. Sophie's mother related that Sophie had always achieved at primary school at just below average, despite apparently good ability. She had found the transfer to secondary school difficult. Her friends from primary school began to distance themselves from her and said they found her 'silly' and 'immature'.

By Year 8, Sophie was reported to have below average attainment with poor concentration and her teacher was describing problems with 'cheeky, disruptive, choice behaviours'. Sophie's parents were concerned that she might have dyslexia and took her for a private assessment. This did not suggest dyslexia but showed that Sophie was in fact of high IQ but that she appeared to have very poor attention skills.

Sophie's parents were prompted further to request referral when they found two empty vodka bottles in her room.

As part of the assessment for possible ADHD a specialist nurse visited school. She observed very poor concentration and impulsive behaviour. She also noted that Sophie spent break times with the boys and behaved in a 'flirtatious' manner towards them. She reported this to Sophie's family.

The day before the next clinic visit Sophie's mother telephones in distress. She has discovered that Sophie has been self-harming. There are shallow cuts on her forearms. Sophie has missed her last period and a pregnancy test is positive.

Suffering in silence

When it comes to age, sex, socioeconomic background, ethnicity or race, ADHD makes no distinction, yet an inherent bias in many referrers' and clinicians' minds skews the diagnostic process towards 'classic' young boy symptoms (restlessness, hyperactivity, inattention and impulsivity), leaving out a significant subgroup of sufferers who do not meet the above classic symptoms: girls of all ages.

Background

A common criticism of the ADHD criteria in the previous Diagnostic and Statistical Manual of Mental Disorders (DSM-IV-TR) in 2000 has been that the core symptoms reflect how the disorder presents in school-age children, and particularly in boys, but do not capture how ADHD presents in older adolescents, some boys, adults and a significant proportion of girls with ADHD. Because of this, some have argued that to reflect the variation in the expression of ADHD, different symptom sets should be developed for different groups.

DSM-5 has tried to address this by making a number of subtle but very important changes to the diagnostic criteria for ADHD (Box 14.1). First, symptoms no longer need to be present by the age of 7 years but by the age of 12 years, thus accounting for those who for a variety of constitutional or environmental factors do not become symptomatic until they enter secondary education or sometimes later. Second, the number of inattentive and hyperactive-impulsive criteria needed to make the diagnosis has been reduced, and the symptoms (rather than impairment) need to be present in two or more settings. Third, although the categories (subtypes) have been retained, they are now referred to as 'presentations' to reflect a desire to move from the more static language of 'subtypes' to a term that better reflects the fluidity and change in how the disorder may present in the same individual over time. All in all, the criteria have become less stringent, and it remains to be seen whether the rates of ADHD diagnoses, particularly in less 'typical' groups such as girls, will increase.

The vast majority of ADHD studies have either been conducted on school-age boys or have included only a few girls and, in particular, very few adolescent girls in the sample. Sex differences in diagnosis were first highlighted in a 1994 National Institute of Mental Health conference (Arnold 1996) followed by a research review (Gaub & Carlson 1997).

In the first large and most comprehensive study of girls with ADHD (Biederman et al. 1999b), 59% were found to have the combined subtype (inattentive and hyperactive/impulsive), only 7% had the predominantly hyperactive/impulsive type, and 27% were found to have the predominantly inattentive subtype. This significant, large, inattentive group of girls is frequently missed early on, with often devastating consequences for their later educational, social and emotional development.

Box 14.1: Relevant changes in DSM-5

✓ Symptoms no longer need to be present by the age of 7 years but by the age of 12

✓ The number of inattentive and hyperactive-impulsive criteria needed to make the diagnosis has been reduced and the symptoms (rather than impairment) need to be present in two or more settings

✓ Categories (subtypes) have been retained but are now referred to as 'presentations' to move from the more static 'subtypes' to a term that better reflects the fluidity in how the disorder may present in different individuals or the same individual over time

---

An early diagnosis and treatment of ADHD is very important as it will lead to better cognitive, academic, social and psychological functioning in subsequent years (Weiss et al. 1985). It therefore becomes crucial that at least by early adolescence those with this condition will have been correctly identified and receiving treatment.

However, evidence suggests that many girls with ADHD are still not recognised. The ratio of school-age boys with ADHD to school-age girls with ADHD is between 6:1 and 12:1 in clinic samples and 3:1 in community samples, but may be equal if the inattentive subtype is considered (Gaub & Carlson 1997). In adult cohorts the ratio is nearer 1:1 male to female. Often, by the time girls are finally suspected of having ADHD and are referred for diagnosis and treatment, the opportunity for early treatment has been missed. They are much older and they have deteriorated so much that their presentation is similar to that of very disturbed, hyperactive boys but with the added complexity of secondary comorbidity.

In this chapter we consider specific issues relating to girls and young women with ADHD.

Presentation and diagnostic issues

Although some girls do present with 'classic' ADHD symptoms, it is vital to also consider an ADHD diagnosis when seeing girls and young women with a variety of other presenting symptoms. As the diagnostic approach for ADHD is biased in favour of disruptive behaviour and male sex (Biederman et al. 1994), girls displaying symptoms of inattention and disorganisation but no conduct problems constitute something other than a variant of ADHD in the minds of their parents, teachers and often clinicians, and are more likely to be thought of as having a learning disability (Hinshaw 2002).

Teachers have often had minimal training about the specific characteristics of ADHD in girls and they may be more reluctant to raise concerns about a girl's poor academic performance and social clumsiness because they are uncertain about the validity of their opinion or are unwilling to 'label' an otherwise well-behaving student, fearing this may lead to embarrassment or stigmatisation (Box 14.2).

Girls, especially those who are actually innately intelligent, are often better able to compensate for their ADHD symptoms in class, particularly in primary school. They may work hard to hide their inattentive symptoms, resulting in less obvious academic difficulties. Girls may be more compliant to teachers' expectations. They are under greater pressure from their parents and teachers to conform to social norms for girls, and they appear more willing to adapt to social demands so as to try to fit in with their peer group.

Girls with the inattentive presentation of ADHD daydream more, and appear passive, academically withdrawn and underachieving. They are often shy, timid and easily overwhelmed. They are more readily distracted and more forgetful, and they lose or misplace their things. They are highly disorganised and they have difficulty following through with tasks and assignments. They rarely act out and they may have difficulty verbalising their thoughts and feelings. They can be easily discouraged and may appear 'sluggish', lazy and lethargic.

Everyday activities overwhelm them. They are often late and poor at timekeeping. They describe feeling different, 'out of tune', unable to function in their peer group, and rejected, with perhaps only one or no friends. They try to remain unnoticed and they easily feel embarrassed and hurt. Their difficulties may result in a sense of shame, self-doubt and

---

Box 14.2: Factors contributing to a lack of recognition/referral of girls with ADHD

ADHD is still thought of as a condition that affects young boys, the cardinal symptom of which is hyperactivity.

Girls:

✓ Are less likely to attract attention by unruly disruptive behaviour

✓ Often work hard to compensate for their ADHD symptoms and present with less obvious academic difficulties

✓ Are more likely to try to comply with and conform to adolescent-group, parental and teacher expectations

✓ Are more prone to be misdiagnosed as anxious or depressed

Teachers may be more reluctant to raise concerns about a girl's poor academic performance and social clumsiness because:

✓ They have had inadequate training about recognising the symptoms of ADHD in girls

✓ Are uncertain about the validity of their opinion

✓ Are unwilling to 'label' an otherwise well-behaved student

inadequacy. At the same time they may display strong and exaggerated feelings when under pressure, hurt or when they feel unjustly criticised.

Social and academic pressures reach a climax in the mass education system of secondary school, which is often ADHD-unfriendly. The school day starts too early, it lasts too long and it demands that students find their way around a large, often complex maze of corridors and staircases in order to get to their various classrooms on time. Pupils are expected to focus, concentrate, be organised and proactive throughout the school day, demands that by far exceed the capacity of most students, even those without ADHD.

Those girls who are particularly bright, resourceful, better adjusted psychologically and who have a nurturing, supportive, encouraging and facilitating family and school environment ('scaffolding') are able to mask and compensate for their ADHD symptoms for longer. This results in a much later diagnosis, at those junctures in life where academic, organisational, social and emotional demands have become overwhelming and are no longer responsive to the supportive structures the girls may have enjoyed up until that time. Typical precipitating milestones are secondary school entry, GCSE/A level or University enrolment.

The challenges of adolescence

Adolescents are victims of the widespread adult belief that adolescence is a transient stage not to be enjoyed in its own right but a passage that prepares for adulthood. The pressure to 'grow up' and become 'responsible' and 'mature' precedes adolescence and increases dramatically with time.

A girl's inattentive ADHD presentation that has not been recognised during her early years is no less real when it emerges during adolescence, a time when the demands for planning, organisation, time management, negotiating social relationships, academic focus and performance become intense, sometimes accompanied by severe, often internalising behaviour disturbance. The changes within DSM-5 begin to recognise this (Box 14.1).

The pressure to conform to the peer group's unwritten and constantly shifting rules and expectations can become the driving force and raison d'être for any adolescent girl. An enormous and disproportionate amount of energy is often spent on analysing and scrutinising their peers: they watch, they comment, they gossip, they compare, they imitate, they identify, they conform, they criticise. However, although in typical adolescent girls this is a developmentally challenging phase they are nevertheless able to negotiate, such activities seem to be more common, frequent and severe and to cause deep despair and despondency in adolescent girls with ADHD.

Girls with ADHD start having social difficulties from their preschool years (Greene et al. 2001), but these particularly impact on them during adolescence when they begin the psychological separation from their family and their social life, and status within their peer group and the formation of early intimate relationships acquire a much greater importance. Many older women with ADHD recall feeling 'different' from the other girls when growing up and being marginalised by their female peer group. The need to overcome this apparent 'difference' and to be accepted by a peer group during teenage years is intense and, in an effort to 'belong', it may lead to dangerous or self-destructive behaviour such as smoking, drinking and unprotected sexual experimentation.

Understanding, acceptance and support from the family is crucial, but it can do little to compensate for the damaging feelings of not belonging and rejection. The peer group is perceived as all-important during adolescence. The low self-esteem and anxiety that adolescent girls with ADHD commonly experience as a result is disturbing, unsettling and will often haunt them for years to come.

Identity confusion, self-doubt, anxiety, uncertainty about the future and insecurity about one's core values are endemic in adolescence. However, the special challenges girls with ADHD face greatly intensify these feelings. Society in general and families in particular have already drawn a 'script' for what they expect of their sons and daughters. For girls, the demands are greater than for boys and they come sooner. For example, girls are encouraged and expected to be dressed 'appropriately', to be 'feminine' (controlled and passive), to emulate older female role models (mothers, teachers), to be carefully presented (in order not to be criticised, something that may reflect on their families), sensitive to the feelings of others (preparation for motherhood), obedient and compliant with adults (submissive). These expectations are very often the direct opposites to the natural tendencies of many girls with ADHD.

Most adolescent girls with ADHD make attempts to comply with these expectations, sometimes obsessively, in an attempt to gain some approval and respect from their family and teachers. However, they often let themselves down in the eyes of their parents by the chaotic state of their rooms and their inability to find the right clothes to wear on school mornings. They may try hard to be fashionable and well dressed, to be part of the 'crowd' and to compensate for the disappointments they experience with their peer group, but they frequently still find themselves unable to gain acceptance from their peers and fail to avoid their sneers and caustic remarks.

In addition to their failure to understand social cues and to meet the demands of social conventions, they also appear to lack both focus and timing in social situations. Janet Giler, in her book (Giler 2000), identifies specific problems in five areas (Box 14.3). Although all of these are important, the issue of poor listening skills is probably most crucial. Listening requires taking the time to let the other person be the centre of attention by focusing on the topic; however, girls with ADHD want to interrupt or change the topic

> **Box 14.3:** Social skills issues for girls with ADHD
>
> Girls with ADHD often struggle in social relationships because they:
>
> ✓ Appear uninterested as a result of poor listening skills and distractability
> ✓ Display poor management of anger and volatile mood swings
> ✓ Appear to brag or be outspoken and seem self-involved
> ✓ Forget appointments or arrive late
> ✓ Appear disinterested in others by not remembering or checking with their friends about their feelings, relationships or reactions to events that have occurred in the friend's life

Source: Adapted from Giler (2000).

and tell how they were affected or reminded of an experience they had. Unfortunately, this makes the adolescent with ADHD the centre of the conversation, often perceived as selfish, self-centred or just uninterested in others. In addition, failure to filter thoughts, being impulsive about someone else's flaws or being over-complimentary about their own abilities, looks or interests can also cause a range of socialisation difficulties.

Anxiety, depression and self-harm

Anxiety and depression often begin during the pressure years of adolescence, and many adolescent girls and later women with ADHD find themselves treated for depression or anxiety, while their ADHD symptoms go unrecognised and untreated (Kessler et al. 2006).

Recent studies have also explored the association between ADHD and deliberate self-harm (DSH) and they reveal that children and young people with ADHD are significantly more likely to deliberately self-harm compared to non-ADHD comparisons, with odds ratios between 4.4 (Hinshaw et al. 2012) and 6.1 (Hurtig et al. 2012). Although the prevalence of females with ADHD presenting with DSH is greater than males (Meza et al. 2015), females with ADHD may be consistently under-identified and under-diagnosed (Gaub & Carlson 1997; Biederman et al. 2002; Quin 2008). Recommendations from these studies suggest there is a need for clinicians to screen for ADHD in those who present with DSH in order to reduce further DSH episodes and potential suicide (Allely 2014).

Emotional reactions and the role of hormones

Most adolescents are 'jumpy', but the typical hyper-sensitivity and hyper-reactivity of ADHD increases during adolescence as hormonal fluctuations complicate and escalate behaviour, often making it unpredictable. The self-doubts, sensitivity to criticism, frailty of feelings, competitiveness, abruptness and irritability so common among adolescent girls are often much more exaggerated in girls with ADHD. They are hurt much more easily, and these painful feelings can have a devastating effect, rapidly escalating into impulsive over-reactions, be they verbal remarks or behaviours including impulsive self-harm. However, as soon as the storm is over they behave as if nothing has happened and they are surprised and bewildered when those they have stung with their comments remain bruised and intolerant of further temper explosions. As far as they are concerned, they have forgotten the incident and forgiven the culprit; perceiving themselves as almost never in the wrong.

Seventy-five per cent of menstruating women experience some premenstrual symptoms with 10% of those being classified as severe and requiring treatment. During that time, ADHD symptoms become magnified with mood instability, disorganisation, forgetfulness, anxiety, depression, fatigue and insomnia being the most prominent.

Sexual activity and risk-taking behaviours

Poor impulse control, restricted thinking of the consequences of one's behaviour and the need to 'belong' may send adolescent girls with ADHD in the direction of early unprotected sexual experimentations and a greater risk for involvement with multiple partners, unwanted pregnancies and sexually transmitted diseases than other adolescent girls (Arnold 1996). Their chronic low self-esteem and the need to be part of a peer group steers them to seek affirmation through the sexual attentions of boys in an effort to compensate for feelings of inadequacy in other areas of their lives.

Substance misuse and addiction risks

Experimentation with alcohol, nicotine and substances begins much earlier in young people with ADHD and adolescent girls are no exception. Sixty per cent of adolescents with ADHD will have used illicit substances by the age of 14 years compared to 17 years for controls; 15% of adolescent girls with ADHD already have a substance use disorder (SUD) and one in five smokes cigarettes (Biederman et al. 1999b). What is even more worrying is that it takes 6 years for 50% of teenagers without ADHD to remit from substance abuse compared with 12 years for patients with ADHD (Wilens et al. 1998). Box 14.4 summarises some issues to consider when assessing girls and young women.

How parents and professionals can help

Box 14.5 lists some issues to consider when supporting young women with ADHD. Once the possibility of ADHD is considered, a specialist assessment is needed to confirm the diagnosis and any comorbid conditions. Computer programs such as the Test of Variables of Attention (TOVA) or the Qb test (Qb tech) (Shirba & Singh 2009) may be

---

Box 14.4: Key learning points to remember when assessing girls and young women with ADHD

- ✓ Remember to consider ADHD when girls and young women present with a wide variety of symptoms (e.g. with possible learning difficulties, poor self-esteem, anxiety, depression, social skills difficulties and self-harm)
- ✓ Hyperactivity is often very small movements such as finger tapping, so difficult to spot
- ✓ Girls who have specifically inattentive profile do not draw attention to themselves and are often difficult to spot
- ✓ Internalising symptoms make girls more vulnerable to low self-esteem, anxiety and mood disorders
- ✓ Girls often have to put in far more effort to keep up performance in line with peers. They then often struggle when increasing social, organisational and learning demands outstrip their ability to compensate with extra effort
- ✓ Social immaturity becomes very apparent alongside other girls in secondary setting, resulting in them being 'dropped from the group' so they may spend more time with boys
- ✓ Flirtatious behaviour may move quickly into impulsive sexual activity
- ✓ Pre-menstrual worsening of ADHD symptoms is common
- ✓ Cutting and self-harming may be the initial presentation of ADHD in girls
- ✓ An overlap with ASD may become more apparent as demand increases

---

Box 14.5: Things to consider in the management of ADHD in girls and young women

- ✓ Careful diagnostic assessment of possible ADHD and comorbid conditions, particularly anxiety, depression and self-harm
- ✓ Psychoeducation specific to the presenting symptoms
- ✓ Psychotherapy specific to the girl/young woman's needs
- ✓ Medication for ADHD and if needed for comorbid conditions
- ✓ Scaffolding support at home and at school

---

helpful in confirming the diagnosis and give a visual demonstration to the young woman and her family and teachers (who may still be sceptical about the ADHD diagnosis).

Treatment begins with the imparting of information and the chance to develop an understanding of the diagnosis. Medication and psychotherapy used together seem to be the most effective ongoing treatment.

A full medical examination should precede any pharmacological treatment. In my experience it is important to consider abnormalities in thyroid function. Hyperthyroidism may correlate with hyperactivity, but not inattention, whereas hypothyroidism can link with affective disorders. Five per cent of the general population and 10% of women suffer from subclinical hypothyroidism associated with subtle deficits in attention and memory, and this may present as a vulnerability to depression.

Stimulants are the treatment of choice, and the response rate in girls is similar to that of boys, but they may increase anxiety in already anxious patients. Atomoxetine may then be successful, or sustained-release guanfacine. Appetite suppression by stimulants may lead to weight loss. Particular care in monitoring is needed if the young woman also has symptoms of anorexia. If the girl/young woman is pregnant, ADHD medications should be avoided during pregnancy, but considered after delivery, especially if she is caring for the baby. Practical support should also be provided.

Medication regimes often need to address a complex set of issues, including anxiety and/or depression, rather than ADHD alone, and in clinical practice some medications for mood disorders may interfere with attention. Comorbid anxiety or depression needs thorough assessment, and careful decisions need to be made as to which disorder needs prior treatment and if both need medication (see Chapter 11).

The intensity of feelings and reactions so often seen in adolescent girls with ADHD has a neurobiological basis and their reactions tend to be even more extreme at times of stress, fatigue, hunger, sleeplessness or premenstrual symptoms (PMS). The adolescent girl's parents and teachers need to recognise the additional vulnerability that she has and begin to identify and manage the potential stresses that can worsen her reactions.

Relationships with peers and issues of self-image and self-worth are so dominant among most adolescent girls with ADHD that psychotherapy needs to be specifically aimed at addressing these. Group psychotherapy can be very supportive and effective, because the group can serve as a platform for sharing experiences and coping strategies with like-minded adolescents, and such groups could take place in school with an experienced school counsellor, or in a community mental health service.

Many mothers are hypercritical of their daughters with ADHD, often through lack of knowledge about the condition. These mother–daughter relationship issues need to be thoroughly addressed, clarified and hopefully resolved either in formal or informal therapy sessions and discussions. ADHD being a highly inherited condition, several mothers will recognise similar symptoms in themselves.

The need for and benefits of external structures

Adolescent girls with ADHD need their family to provide them with structure, support and encouragement in order to maintain some order in their lives, something that most parents try to do, unless they themselves have similar organisational difficulties. However, during adolescence and in their quest for independence and gradual separation from their parents, it is probably wiser if someone other than the parents provides this structure if possible. This can be a therapist, a coach, a school counsellor or a trusted relative who will be discreet and maintain confidentiality. Learning to be on time, developing strategies to improve organisation, setting priorities and being proactive rather than staying in a reactive mode, must be seen as being for their benefit and not as something imposed by their parents.

Despite their critical stance towards many of their elders, adolescents look up to role models to help them further discover and develop their self-identity, self-awareness and confidence and to sharpen those skills necessary to assert themselves and negotiate peer relationships for independent living beyond the school.

Focus on positive attributes and strengths

Those who have a talent or ability they can apply constructively are better protected from the brooding of boredom, self-pity and dejection. Schools can play a big part in helping girls with ADHD through their secondary years by actively encouraging and helping them discover, recognise, develop and apply areas of competence and talent. The more they are aware and proud of their skills and talents, the less likely they are to fall victim to criticisms and frustrations. Many secondary schools facilitate activities such as involvement in after-school charitable events, voluntary work or taking part in community projects. Involving adolescent girls with ADHD in well-structured, constructive and rewarding activities may help them channel their creative energies, increase their confidence and help them improve their sense of self-worth. Recent studies confirm what we have always known, that those adolescents who are kept out of harm's way, busy with extracurricular activities, sports, and so on, are less likely to get into trouble during secondary school (Guindon 2009).

Treatment of premenstrual syndrome

Premenstrual syndrome (PMS), premenstrual tension (PMT) or premenstrual dysphoric disorder (PMDD) particularly affect adolescent girls with ADHD. Oestrogen has been known to have a profound effect on mood, mental state and memory by activating monoamine and neurotransmitter mechanisms and stimulating dopamine D-2 receptors in the striatum. During the low-oestrogen premenstrual part of their cycle, many young women experience low frustration tolerance, irritability, anxiety, memory deficits, confusion, sleep disturbance, depression and panic, but those with ADHD will experience these at a much greater intensity that may require immediate and active intervention.

Clinicians involved in managing adolescent girls with ADHD should be aware of this additional vulnerability and remain up to date on research on PMS and new treatment approaches. Selective serotonin re-uptake inhibitors (SSRIs) are well known to control PMS, and more recent research suggests, in addition, low-dose contraception (progestin drospirenone), oestrogen patches and implants, gonadotrophin-releasing hormone (GnRH) analogues or analgesics (Rapkin & Winer 2008) may be helpful.

Treatment of anxiety and depression

When everything around the already stressed and strained adolescent girl with ADHD appears to be overwhelming, emotions can easily and rapidly flare up and become uncontrollable. The fall out with one or more of her peers, the rejection and exclusion from her peer group, the break-up of a relationship, ongoing arguments with her parents, a failed exam, a university entrance rejection – any of these is enough to push her into depths of anxiety or depression.

Vigilance by all involved is paramount during these years in order to evaluate whether these are more likely to be ordinary emotional adolescent fluctuations or whether the adolescent with ADHD has developed frank anxiety or depression that requires treatment in its own right in conjunction with ADHD medication. Because stimulants for ADHD may increase anxiety, changing to atomoxetine may be considered or a small dose of an antidepressant may effectively counteract anxiety and also treat depressive symptoms.

Self-harm, including attempted suicide, is a significantly higher risk in this group. Families, teachers and clinicians need to be aware and respond to low mood promptly and assess carefully (see also Chapter 11).

Sexual risk counselling

Sex education in schools from an early age addresses the risks associated with sexual behaviour, but specific groups for adolescent girls with ADHD could help them feel more accepted and less alone and therefore less prone to seek male sexual attention. An open, genuine, trusting, honest and supportive relationship with their parents gives them somewhere to turn to for advice if they become sexually active, either to help them make a sensible choice of birth control or to help them make the best decision they can should they accidentally become pregnant. A holistic approach in ADHD services should also enable girls and young women to discuss issues around sexual health and contraception with other trusted adults and, if necessary, inform them and their families about other helpful local resources.

Summary

- Despite numerous discussions around the need to have sex-based diagnostic criteria for ADHD, mental health professionals continue to rely on behaviour criteria that better identify disruptive boys. As a result, ADHD in young girls often remains unrecognised and usually presents later and with internalising rather than externalising symptoms.

- Health professionals, teachers and society as a whole need to be aware that ADHD often presents differently in girls and young women and be proactive in seeking assessment and treatment if appropriate.

- The adolescent years are especially challenging for teenage girls with ADHD. They need their parents and teachers to acknowledge and be informed of their condition, to provide support and guidance while respecting the adolescent's need for developing autonomy.

- Appropriate medical and psychological treatment should be provided, depending on their particular circumstances, needs and issues.

- Given the right support and timely interventions, they can master this transition from the confusion and self-doubt to a sense of developing self-awareness, inner strength, self-esteem as they enter their young adult years.

References

Allely CS (2014) The association of ADHD symptoms to self-harm behaviours: a systematic PRISMA review. *BMC Psychiatry* 14(1): 133.

American Psychiatric Association (2000) *Diagnostic and statistical manual of mental disorders,* 4th edn. Washington, DC: American Psychiatric Association.

American Psychiatric Association (2013) *Diagnostic and statistical manual of mental disorders,* 5th edn. Washington, DC: American Psychiatric Association.

Arnold LE (1996) Sex differences in AD/HD: Conference summary. *J Abn Child Psychol* 24(5): 555–569.

Biederman J, Faraone SV, Spencer T et al. (1994) Gender differences in a sample of adults with attention deficit hyperactivity disorder. *Psychiatry Res* 53: 13–29.

Biederman J, Wilens T, Mick E et al. (1999a) Pharmacotherapy of attention deficit/hyperactivity disorder reduces risk for substance use disorder. *Pediatrics* 104: e20.

Biederman J, Faraone SV, Mick E et al. (1999b) Clinical correlates of AD/HD in females: Findings from a large group of girls ascertained from pediatric and psychiatric referral sources. *J Am Acad Child Adolesc Psychiatry* 38(8): 966–975.

Biederman, J, Mick, E, Faraone SV et al. (2002) Influence of gender on attention deficit hyperactivity disorder in children referred to a psychiatric clinic. *Am J Psychiatry* 159: 36–42.

Gaub M, Carlson CL (1997) Gender differences in AD/HD: A meta-analysis and critical review. *J Am Acad Child Adolesc Psychiatry* 36: 1036–1045.

Giler J (2000) *Socially Addept: A manual for parents of children with ADHD and/or learning disabilities.* CES Continuing Education Seminars.

Greene RW, Biederman J, Faraone SV et al. (2001) Social impairment in girls with AD/HD: Patterns, gender comparisons, and correlates. *J Am Acad Child Adolesc Psychiatry* 40: 704–710.

Guindon M (ed.) (2009) *Self-esteem across the lifespan.* Routledge, New York, NY.

Hinshaw SP (2002) Preadolescent girls with attention deficit/hyperactivity disorder: I. Background characteristics, comorbidity, cognitive and social functioning and parenting practices. *J Consult Clin Psychol* 70: 1086–1098.

Hinshaw SP, Owens EB, Zalecki C et al. (2012) Prospective follow-up of girls with attention-deficit/ hyperactivity disorder into early adulthood: Continuing impairment includes elevated risk for suicide attempts and self-injury. *J Consult Clin Psychol* 80(6): 1041.

Hurtig T, Taanila A, Moilanen I, Nordström T, Ebeling H (2012) Suicidal and self-harm behaviour associated with adolescent attention deficit hyperactivity disorder – a study in the Northern Finland Birth Cohort 1986. *Nordic J Psychiatry* 66(5): 320–328.

Kessler RC, Adler L, Barkley R et al. (2006) The prevalence and correlates of adult AD/HD in the United States: Results from the national comorbidity survey replication. *Am J Psychiatry* 163: 716–723.

Meza JI, Owens EB, Hinshaw SP (2015) Response inhibition, peer preference and victimization, and self-harm: Longitudinal associations in young adult women with and without ADHD. *J Abnorm Child Psychol* 2015: 1–12.

Quinn PO (2008) Attention-deficit/hyperactivity disorder and its comorbidities in women and girls: An evolving picture. *Curr Psychiatry Rep* 10(5): 419–423.

Rapkin A, Winer S (2008) The pharmacologic management of premenstrual dysphoric disorder. *Exp Opin Pharmacother* 9(3): 429–445.

Sharma A, Singh B (2009) Evaluation of the role of QB testing in attention deficit hyperactivity disorder. *Arch Dis Child* 94: A72.

Weiss G, Hechtman L, Milroy T, Perlman T (1985) Psychiatric status of hyperactives as adults: A controlled prospective 15-year follow-up of 63 hyperactive children. *J Am Acad Child Psychiatry* 24: 211–220.

Wilens T, Biederman J, Mick E (1998) Does AD/HD affect the course of substance abuse? Findings from a sample of adults with and without AD/HD. *Am J Addict* 7(2): 156–163.

Chapter 15

ADHD and substance misuse in young people

KAH Mirza, Sudeshni Mirza and Roshin M Sudesh

Introduction

Substance misuse is one of the most common public health problems in adolescence. Many young people who engage in the misuse of drugs and alcohol have multiple antecedent and coexisting mental health problems, and substance misuse takes a high toll in terms of healthcare costs, violent crime, accidents, suicide, social and interpersonal difficulties, and educational impairment (Mirza et al. 2011). In Europe, the prevalence of alcohol misuse is high, with up to 90% of students aged 15 or 16 years having consumed alcohol and, on average, 21% of boys and 15% of girls having tried illicit drugs at least once. About 38% of young people report that they have engaged in 'heavy, episodic drinking' (binge drinking, defined as consuming five or more drinks per occasion) during the past 30 days (European School Survey Project on Alcohol and Other Drugs (ESPAD) 2015, reported in Hibell et al. 2009). According to the 2013 British Crime Survey (Home Office 2014), 16.3% of young people aged 16–24 years had taken an illicit drug in the last year, and the lifetime use of illicit drugs was 36.7%. Tobacco, alcohol and cannabis were the most commonly abused substances, with cocaine and heroin accounting for less than 10% (Home Office 2014; ESPAD 2015).

ADHD is a common, heterogeneous neuropsychiatric condition that can persist into adolescence (Taylor et al. 1996) and adulthood (Biederman et al. 2006). Over the past decade, a robust body of evidence has emerged to indicate that the overlap between substance misuse and ADHD is larger than expected by chance (Mirza et al. 2012).

Clinicians trying to help people who have both problems face many uncertainties. It is often unclear how an individual should be assessed and advised, and what forms of treatment should be offered. Specialist services for one condition sometimes exclude the other. National guidelines appear to be lacking. As ADHD is a risk factor for the development of substance misuse, clinicians would be helped by a secure knowledge of the developmental pathways involved in the transition from ADHD to substance misuse so that they could develop early-targeted interventions to prevent substance misuse.

This chapter aims to bring together information about the comorbidity of ADHD and substance misuse and to make clinical recommendations about managing the combination of problems. We shall use the term 'substance misuse' throughout this chapter to refer to problematic substance use, including harmful use and substance dependence as described by the International Classification of Disorders (WHO 1993). The term 'substance misuse' as used in the UK is roughly equivalent to substance use disorder as described in the 5th edition of the Diagnostic and Statistical Manual of Disorders (American Psychiatric Association 2013). However, adult classification systems are inadequate in capturing the developmental stages of substance use in young people and may potentially prevent earlier interventions in young people who are at risk of developing severe forms of substance misuse in late adolescence or adulthood (Gilvarry et al. 2012).

How common is substance misuse in ADHD and ADHD in substance misuse?

Prospective, longitudinal follow-up studies conducted in community samples and clinical populations show that children with ADHD are at high risk of developing substance misuse (Barkley et al. 2004; Biederman et al. 2006). A recent meta-analysis of 27 longitudinal studies that prospectively followed children with ADHD into adolescence and adulthood showed that children with ADHD have a 1.5-fold increase in risk of developing any substance misuse and nearly three times higher risk for nicotine dependence than those without ADHD (Lee et al. 2011). Another meta-analytic study of 13 follow-up studies (Charach et al. 2011) showed that childhood ADHD was associated with alcohol misuse by young adulthood and with nicotine misuse by middle adolescence. The risk, however, may be due to other influences besides ADHD itself, such as coexisting conduct disorder or social adversity.

Conversely, studies in adolescent and adult populations attending substance misuse clinics have shown that between 20% and 30% have concomitant ADHD (Levin et al. 1998; Schubiner et al. 2000). Patients with both ADHD and substance misuse become dependent on substances at a younger age, use more substances and are hospitalised more often than substance misusing patients without ADHD (Arias et al. 2008). Persistent ADHD affects the onset, course and prognosis of substance misuse in adolescents and adults (see Mirza & Buckstein 2010 for a review).

Why and how does the association arise?

Developmental pathways involved in the transition from ADHD to substance misuse

The relationship between ADHD and substance misuse is complex and unlikely to reflect a single pathway. The possible reasons for the strong associations between ADHD and substance misuse may be direct or could be artefactual (e.g. resulting from the close link between ADHD and conduct disorders). This has implications for clinical input (Box 15.1).

Box 15.1: Possible reasons for the strong associations between ADHD and substance misuse

Possible cause for association	Strength of evidence	Clinical implications
Prenatal exposure to nicotine and possibly alcohol increase risk of development of ADHD →	Strong evidence for the role of nicotine use, less so for alcohol use →	Primary prevention efforts aimed at reducing maternal smoking during pregnancy
ADHD leads to substance misuse through the development of conduct disorders →	Strong evidence, especially if social adversity coexists →	Prevention efforts should involve detection and management of conduct disorders by offering psychological treatments
ADHD increases the risk for substance misuse – especially for nicotine dependence →	Evidence is equivocal →	Regular monitoring and preventive efforts to reduce the risk of development of nicotine dependence
Potential for ADHD medications to cause misuse of themselves or other substances →	No evidence so far to suggest increased risk, but diversion and misuse is possible →	Active treatment of ADHD is indicated, even if substance misuse coexists. Take steps to prevent diversion and misuse of stimulants
The effects of shared common causes such as genetic/neurobiological influences or psychosocial variables such as social deprivation →	Evidence so far is equivocal at this stage →	Public policy and prevention should pay more attention to address the putative risk factors
Self-medication hypothesis →	Very little evidence →	Active treatment of ADHD should reduce the risk of further misuse

A detailed analysis of the existing literature about the causal pathways and mechanisms of association between ADHD and substance misuse is beyond the scope of this chapter, and interested readers may refer to reviews by Mirza and Taylor (forthcoming). We shall, however, try to address one of the major questions that exercise clinicians at the coalface reality of clinical practice: does prescription of stimulants for ADHD increase the risk of substance misuse?

Are we at risk of doing more harm than good?

Review of evidence

Pharmacotherapy is a central component of interventions in children with ADHD, and there is a robust body of evidence to attest to the efficacy and safety of stimulants, and other drugs, at least in the short term (NICE 2006). Over the previous two decades there has been a substantial increase in recognition of the disorder and a corresponding rise in the number of children and young people treated with stimulant medication. In the UK, the numbers rose from an estimated 0.5/1000 children diagnosed 30 years ago to more than 3/1000 receiving medication in the late 1990s (NICE 2008). Epidemiological data from the UK database revealed a trend of increasing prescribing prevalence of ADHD drug treatment over the period 2003–2008 overall and for all age groups (McCarthy et al. 2012). However the numbers treated are much lower than published estimates of the prevalence of ADHD. Concerns have been expressed from a number of quarters regarding the exponential rise in the prescription of medications to control behaviour (Timimi 2002) and in particular about the potential risk of substance misuse as a result of prescribing stimulants to treat ADHD (Robbins 2002).

We shall aim to address this controversy by exploring the evidence from animal, clinical and pharmacological studies, followed by the clinical implications.

Animal studies

A large number of studies in rats have shown that methylphenidate, when administered parenterally, is quite similar to cocaine and amphetamine in terms of its reinforcing properties. At this stage, the data from animal studies regarding sensitisation are conflicting at best, and it is difficult to extrapolate the findings to human beings, for a variety of reasons (see Kollins et al. 2001 for a comprehensive review of animal studies). There are no well-designed studies to address this issue in human beings, so it is difficult to reliably answer the question 'Does early exposure to stimulant medication lead to sensitisation to stimulants or other drugs in later life?'

Pharmacological studies

All drugs of abuse act by increasing dopamine in the mesolimbic and mesocortical dopamine pathways (Robbins & Everett 2002). Like cocaine, stimulants used for the management of ADHD exert their pharmacological properties by blocking dopamine reuptake, thereby increasing synaptic dopamine. Some studies have shown that methylphenidate is even more potent than cocaine in binding to the dopamine transporter and producing long-lasting neuronal adaptation in the nucleus accumbens (Kollins et al. 2001). Studies with healthy human volunteers have shown that the subjective effects of intravenous methylphenidate are quite similar to those of cocaine and amphetamine (see Kollins et al. 2001 for a comprehensive review). However, seminal studies by Volkow and colleagues from the National Institute of Drug Abuse have shown that the route of administration and dosages of stimulants are the most important variables that determine abuse potential (Volkow & Swanson 2003). When methylphenidate is administered intravenously, it enters the brain like cocaine and peaks rapidly, producing subjective sensations of euphoria. However, when methylphenidate is taken orally, the rate of uptake into the striatum is much slower, and subjective sensations of euphoria are significantly reduced or absent. Similarly, regardless of the routes of administration, methylphenidate is cleared from the body more slowly than cocaine, which may diminish the reinforcing properties and protect against repeated self-administration and misuse (Volkow & Swanson 2003). Thus, methylphenidate, when taken orally in therapeutic doses and within a clinical context, appears to be associated with a much lower abuse potential than cocaine.

Clinical studies

Randomised controlled studies of stimulant therapy thus far have not been long enough to determine any effect on later substance misuse. However, longitudinal community studies and naturalistic studies (which use the methodology of observing a subject's unaltered behaviour in his/her normal environment, without intervention) have followed children diagnosed with ADHD into adolescence or adulthood. A meta-analysis of prospective and retrospective studies conducted up to 2003 reported that those who had been treated with stimulants were protected against the development of substance-related problems (odds ratio of 1.9) compared with those who had not been treated in this way (Wilens et al. 2003). It is hard to be certain about which components of treatment were responsible – whether it was a direct effect of stimulants or the associated aspects of therapy. Interestingly, another recent meta-analysis of 15 studies published between January 1980 and February 2012 based on 2565 participants found that treatment of ADHD with stimulants neither protected nor increased the risk of later substance misuse (Humphreys et al. 2013).

Lambert and colleagues have argued that childhood ADHD and stimulant treatment is related significantly to rates of tobacco use and dependence and cocaine dependence (Lambert 2002). More recently, however, four prospective longitudinal studies have concluded that early stimulant treatment for ADHD does not contribute to substance misuse later in life and that, in fact, methylphenidate may delay the onset of continuous nicotine use (Manuzza et al. 2008; Biederman et al. 2008; Huss et al. 2008; Wilens et al. 2011).

A large-scale, 14-month randomised trial of intensive behavioural therapy against carefully crafted medication has reported on the naturalistic outcome (i.e. measured without offering any systematic interventions during the follow-up period) after the end of randomisation (Molina et al. 2007). At the 36-month point, those who had initially been assigned to behaviour therapy showed a substantial reduction in substance use compared with treatment as usual; medication alone did not appear to affect substance use one way or the other. There is some evidence to suggest that early age at initiation of treatment with methylphenidate in children with ADHD may have beneficial long-term effects on later substance abuse (Manuzza et al. 2008). Similarly, an 8-year follow up of the above National Institute of Mental Health Collaborative Multimodal Treatment Study of Children with ADHD (MTA Study) reported that medication for ADHD did not 'protect from, or contribute to, visible risk of substance use or substance misuse by adolescence', whether analysed as randomised treatment assignment in childhood, as medication at follow-up, or as cumulative stimulant treatment (Molina et al. 2013). Rates of substance use at all time points, including the use of two or more substances and substance misuse, were each higher in the ADHD than in the non-ADHD samples, regardless of sex.

A recent study based on a large-scale nationwide psychiatric cohort of ADHD patients of all ages diagnosed and treated in Denmark (n=20 742) investigated the risk of various medications including stimulants in comparison to a control group of non-medicated patients with ADHD (Steinhausen & Bisgaard 2013). The rates of substance misuse were higher in the non-medicated group, and treatment with stimulants did not increase the risk of substance misuse.

Clinical implications

What clinicians will want to take from the above brief overview is that children and young people who have been diagnosed with ADHD with coexisting conduct disorder are at significant risk for developing substance misuse, and prevention of this developmental path should be included as a routine goal of management. At least a substantial amount of the risk is mediated by the conduct problems (and/or the social adversity leading to them), thus suggesting that reduction of conduct problems and social adversity could be helpful in reducing the risk. The effect of behavioural therapy (in the MTA study) supports the inclusion of psychological and social measures in the long-term treatment of ADHD.

Even those with ADHD without conduct disorder are at considerable risk for cigarette smoking and possibly for other types of substance misuse, not least because they may develop conduct disorder later, again supporting the need for multimodal treatment of ADHD.

As stimulant medication does not appear to increase the risk of substance misuse, its use is not contraindicated. However, the lack of evidence for a self-medication theory of substance use, except perhaps for nicotine, does not support the idea that risk for misuse is in itself an indication for 'preventive' use of stimulant medication.

Diversion and misuse of stimulant medication

Stimulant medications are controlled drugs and have themselves the potential for misuse and diversion, either for subjective euphoric effects or for effects on performance. Methylphenidate can be misused intranasally by crushing the tablets and snorting the powder or intravenously by dissolving the powder in water for injection. People who take the drug to induce euphoria prefer intranasal and intravenous routes, and there have been a few case reports of intravenous abuse of methylphenidate in young adults (Parran & Jasinsky 1991). Extended-release preparations of stimulants are less easy to misuse in this way than immediate-release tablets. More commonly, oral stimulants are misused to enhance performance in sports or some kinds of cognitive tasks and examinations (Wilens et al. 2008). A national survey of 10 904 college students in the USA reported that 4.1% of students had used stimulants for non-medical purposes in the past year, and 54% of students with ADHD on medication had been approached to divert their medication (sell, trade or give away) in the past year (McCabe et al. 2005). Although systematic information regarding the extent of diversion and misuse across the UK is not available, a study conducted in Wirrall, Merseyside, indicated that diversion was common, and the lifetime prevalence of illicit methylphenidate use in young people (31%) was second only to cannabis (Woolfall 2006). Another survey from the same area showed that pharmaceutical preparations of stimulants such as methylphenidate and dexamphetamine were available on the illicit market for as little as 30 pence a tablet (Geraghty 2008).

In summary, prescribed stimulants may be misused through multiple routes, including oral, intravenous and intranasal. In view of the risk of misuse and diversion of stimulant medication, caution should be exercised in the choice of medication, taking into account any personal and family history of substance misuse.

Guidelines for assessment and practical management

Young people presenting with substance misuse and ADHD pose significant challenges for assessment and treatment.

How to recognise and address substance misuse in patients with ADHD?
Children and adolescents with ADHD should be comprehensively assessed for substance misuse, but unfortunately many clinicians working in Paediatrics and Child and Adolescent Mental Health Services do not currently routinely screen young people for

substance misuse (Mirza et al. 2007). Defining substance misuse in young people is not easy. International classificatory systems such as the International Classification of Diseases (ICD-10; WHO 1993) and DSM-5 lack a developmental perspective in psychopathology, and categories such as 'harmful use', 'dependence' and 'substance use disorder' do not seem to capture all stages of substance use in young people (Mirza 2002). Based on the seminal work by Joseph Nowinski (1990), Mirza and Mirza (2008) and Mirza et al. (2011) proposed a developmentally sensitive and dimensional model to classify the stages of substance use in young people, starting with non-use, moving through stages of experimental, social, at-risk (prodromal) and harmful use, to substance dependence (Table 15.1). The above model has the potential to ascertain stages of substance use across the dynamic continuum and help clinicians choose the most appropriate intervention to suit the stage of substance misuse. Naturalistic follow-up studies show that a substantial minority of children who do not meet full criteria for substance misuse are at 'high risk' of developing harmful use/dependence during late adolescence or adulthood (Kandel 2002). From a clinical perspective, it is important to intervene at an early stage, before they have developed entrenched patterns of substance misuse, and the above classification offers a pragmatic choice. Readers may refer to the UK Practice Standards for the assessment and treatment of young people with substance misuse (Gilvarry et al. 2012) for more information.

Young people should be seen separately for a confidential interview. The attitude of the clinician should be flexible, empathic and non-judgmental in order to engage the young person in the assessment process and to obtain a valid estimate of their stage of substance misuse. Clinical and research experience shows that young people are generally more reliable than might be assumed, in terms of the information they can provide regarding substance misuse (Mirza et al. 2011). Explore the young person's leisure-time activities and gently guide them to talk about the nature and extent of substance use, context and impact on various domains of their psychosocial functioning. Detailed exploration of comorbid psychiatric disorders, other risk-taking behaviour and their relationship to substance misuse will help in formulating a differential diagnosis and treatment plan. Specific questions should be asked to determine whether the young person has used another person's drugs, given or sold medication to others, or increased the dosage of a drug without conferring with the doctors. Substance misuse is almost always not the only problem for most young people, and so a comprehensive developmental, social and medical history is a part of any complete assessment. Particular attention should be paid to the young person's vulnerability, resilience, hopes and aspirations. Evaluating the young person's readiness for treatment or stage of change (Di Clemente et al. 2004) may help to determine the initial treatment goals or level of care.

It is important to take a detailed family history, ideally with the help of a genogram, to determine whether there is substance misuse in biological relatives or other family members. Detailed information relating to peer group, including membership or affiliation of the young person to delinquent peer groups, should also be explored.

Specific treatment of substance misuse

Treatment modalities used in substance misuse are largely psychosocial. Although abstinence should remain the explicit long-term goal of treatment, harm reduction may be an interim, implicit goal of treatment, in view of both the chronicity of substance misuse in some young people and the self-limiting nature of substance misuse in others. Comprehensive treatment packages usually consist of individual, group and family/systemic therapies (Williams & Chang 2000). Medication should only be used as an adjunct. However, medication may offer a window of opportunity for young people to engage in psychosocial treatment (Mirza 2002, Marshall & Mirza 2007). Family therapy approaches, such as Multi-Systemic Therapy, Functional Family Therapy and Multidimensional Family Therapy, have the best evidence base for efficacy across a number of domains (Corless et al. 2009), although individual approaches such as cognitive behavioural therapy, either alone or in combination with motivational enhancement, have been shown to be efficacious as well (Waldron & Kaminer 2004). It has been shown that a single session of motivational interviewing (MI) can reduce the use of cigarettes, alcohol and cannabis in young people aged 16–20 years (McCambridge & Strang 2004). Clinicians should try to create links with local Substance Misuse Teams and aim to develop pathways of care to deliver comprehensive treatment for young people with ADHD and substance misuse (Gilvarry et al. 2012).

How can ADHD in patients with substance misuse be recognised and addressed?

The characteristic symptoms of impulsiveness, over activity and inattention can be elicited as in any assessment for ADHD. However, it is important to bear in mind that the clinical picture in adolescents with ADHD, whether they are misusing drugs or not, will show pathoplastic effects of age, and particular attention should be paid to emotional dysregulation, disorganisation and other executive function deficits. Screening questionnaires, informant interviews around past and current functioning, and school information remain relevant. In addition, it is necessary to gain a detailed history of the use of prescribed and recreational drugs. Some drugs (such as cannabis) can bring about inattentiveness, high-dose stimulants can produce marked over-activity (especially of a rather stereotyped form), and cocaine can produce a volatile emotional state. Clinical assessment therefore needs to establish whether the ADHD-type features preceded substance misuse, whether they are trait-like rather than episodic, and whether they have the characteristically disorganised quality of ADHD. Information from people who know the patient well, and knew them in childhood, is crucial for a reliable diagnosis. Repeated assessments may have to be carried out to clarify the diagnosis of ADHD once the substance misuse is stabilised or reduced, through specific interventions for substance misuse.

How should ADHD be treated in the presence of substance misuse?

Integrated, multimodal treatment of both substance misuse and ADHD has been found to be useful in clinical practice (Riggs et al. 2011; Mirza & Buckstein 2010), and specific

Table 15.1 Stages of substance (alcohol and drugs) use and suggested interventions: a pragmatic classification (Mirza & Mirza 2008; Mirza et al. 2011; Gilvarry et al. 2012)

Stage	Motive	Setting	Frequency	Emotional impact	Behaviour	Impact on functioning	Suggested interventions (Gilvarry 2000)
Experimental stage	Curiosity and risk taking	Alone or with peer group	Rarely or very occasionally	Effect of drugs is usually very short term	No active drug-seeking behaviour	Relatively little; may rarely result in dangerous consequences	Universal prevention (drug education, formal or informal)
Social stage	Social acceptance/the need to fit in	Usually with peer group	Occasionally	Mind altering effects of drugs are clearly recognised	No active drug-seeking behaviour	Usually no significant problems, but some can go on to show features of the early at-risk stage	Universal prevention (drug education, formal or informal)
Early at-risk stage	Social acceptance/peer pressure	Facilitated by peer group	Frequent, but variable, depending on peer group	Mind altering effects of drugs are clearly recognised and sought	No active drug-seeking behaviour, but develops a regular pattern of drug/alcohol use	Associated with significant dangers including recurrent binge drinking or problems associated with intoxication	*Targeted intervention/ treatment by non-specialist services (e.g. GP, school health worker, young people's counselling services, healthcare staff working in Child and Adolescent Mental Health Services (CAMHS), Paediatrics, etc.)

Table 15.1 (Continued)

Stage							
Later at-risk stage (substance use is not dominating mental state)	Cope with negative emotions or enhance pleasure	Alone or with a like-minded peer group	Frequent/regular use	Uses drugs to alter mood or behaviour	Active drug-seeking behaviour is a key indicator of this stage	May be impairment in functioning in some areas (e.g. school and family)	Treatment by specialist services (e.g. CAMHS), for both mental health issues and progression of substance use to further serious stages
Stage of harmful use (similar to ICD-10)	Drug use is the primary means of recreation, coping with stress or both	Alone or with an altered (drug using) peer group	Regular use, despite negative consequences	Negative effects on emotions and ability to function	Active drug-seeking behaviour, despite negative consequences across many areas of life	Impairment in almost all areas of life and/or distress within families or close relationships	*Treatment by specialist services (e.g. specialist substance misuse treatment services for young people and specialist substance misuse professionals within CAMHS)
Stage of dependence (similar to ICD-10; only a rare minority of young people progress to this stage)	To deal with withdrawal symptoms, and stop craving	Alone or with like-minded peer group	Compulsive, regular or often daily use to manage withdrawal symptoms	Emotional impacts of drugs are very significant; withdrawal symptoms prominent	Active drug seeking behaviour, often loss of control over use, pre-occupation with drug use, craving, and behaviour may involve criminality	Physical and psychological complications, impairment in all areas of life	*Treatment by specialist services including Detoxification and for some residential rehabilitation

*For some the involvement of agencies and services, other than substance misuse services, may be required.

Source: Modified and reproduced with permission from Mirza & Mirza (2008).

treatment for ADHD and substance misuse should ideally be provided under the same roof. Psychological treatment involving behavioural approaches and parental involvement has a strong place in the treatment of most people with ADHD (NICE 2008) and should also be available to young people using substances. Objective rating scales should be used whenever possible, to document improvement in target symptoms and adaptive functioning.

The most common drugs misused by young people include tobacco, alcohol and cannabis, and only a small proportion of young people use cocaine, heroin or ecstasy. Although abstinence is ideal prior to initiating medication treatment for ADHD, achieving complete or sustained abstinence may not be a realistic expectation for many young people, especially if they suffer from a coexisting untreated psychiatric illness. In practice, once the substance misuse (in the case of misuse of alcohol, cannabis and tobacco) is stabilised through harm-reductions strategies, it is reasonable to commence medication and other treatments for ADHD.

Interactions between drugs we prescribe and they 'prescribe'
Unfortunately, there is very little empirical data to inform clinical practice regarding the interaction between stimulant medication and drugs of misuse. The presence of alcohol or cannabis consumption is not a contraindication to stimulant prescribing, although clinicians should warn young people about the increased risk of side effects if they take alcohol and stimulants together. Concomitant cannabis and stimulant use should be closely monitored in those with a family history or past history of psychosis.

Misuse of cocaine and other stimulants
Although there is little empirical evidence to guide practice in those misusing cocaine and amphetamines (including methamphetamine), the similarity of the mechanism of action of the two drugs (inhibition of the dopamine transporter), albeit with different time courses, suggests that there could be particular dangers in the combination. Hence, such substance misuse, especially if it is chaotic as is often the case with regular amphetamine or cocaine misuse, should be addressed before initiating ADHD medications.

Misuse of opiates
The small minority of young people who present with opiate dependence often live chaotic lifestyles and tend to use a number of drugs other than opiates. It would be prudent to address the issues related to opiate dependence and other psychosocial issues first, before commencing medications for the treatment of ADHD. Stimulants can be used in conjunction with methadone or buprenorphine maintenance programmes, ideally in the context of a comprehensive psychosocial treatment programme to address their multiple complex needs.

Novel psychoactive substances (the so-called 'legal highs')
There is little empirical data to guide clinical practice, when young people are using the new psychoactive substances (NPSs, historically called 'legal highs') such as mephadrone or synthetic cannabinoids (spice), which are easily available through head shops and

the Internet. There is little information on the pharmacology, toxicology and safety of NPSs for humans. They can differ markedly in terms of their ingredients, potency, formulation and harmful effects, so the potential health implications of these compounds are largely unknown. In October 2015, the UK Government issued a blanket ban on all new NPSs. A pragmatic approach in managing comorbid ADHD and NPS misuse may involve addressing the misuse of these drugs first using principles of motivational interviewing and harm minimisation strategies and encouraging the young people to abstain from the NPS while they are receiving ADHD medications, in view of the scientific unknowns about the interactions between the above drugs. For up-to-date information about NPSs, see www.rednetproject.eu.

Evidence base for treatment of young people with ADHD and substance misuse
Although several medications including bupropion have been evaluated in open-label studies in adolescents with ADHD and substance misuse, there are only four published controlled trials (Table 15.2). In summary, although there is too little empirical data to assert the efficacy of medication in adolescents with ADHD and coexisting substance misuse, medication, including stimulants, appears to be safe and does not worsen substance misuse in the short term.

Beyond evidence base: The art and science of creating practice-based evidence
As we have seen so far, there is at present very little empirical evidence to guide treatment for coexisting ADHD and substance misuse. Creativity and a systemic perspective are

Table 15.2 Controlled trials of medications in young people with ADHD and substance misuse

Authors	No. of participants	Medication	Duration of trial	Results	Comments
Riggs et al. (2004)	69	Pemoline	12 weeks	Pemoline superior to placebo	Rare but serious hepatotoxicity
Szobot et al. (2008)	16	Long-acting MPH (MPH–SODAS)	6 weeks	Methyl phenidate superior to placebo	Small sample size, single blind trial
Thurstone et al. (2010)	70	Atomoxetine	12 weeks	ATX group not superior to placebo	Both groups received manualised MI/CBT*
Riggs et al. (2011)	360 (multicentre trial)	OROS-methyl phenidate	12 weeks	OROS-MPH group not superior to placebo	Both groups received manualised MI/CBT*

*MI/CBT: combination of motivational interviewing and cognitive behaviour therapy (CBT) throughout the 12-week trial, which addressed substance misuse.

essential to provide a treatment programme tailored to address the multiple complex needs that many such young people have. Clinicians should work to engage the 'hard to reach' young people in treatment (Box 15.2).

In our experience, creative use of motivational interviewing-based strategies such as exploring 'what is good and not so good about the drugs you prescribe and 'we prescribe' have helped break the ice and develop a collaborative relationship with young people (Boxes 15.3 and 15.4). An individualistic and flexible approach to prescribing has also been found to be helpful. For example, we have prescribed long-acting methylphenidate to young people who, following a period of intensive individual psychological treatment, have cut down their cannabis use to one or two nights per week (i.e. Fridays and Saturdays). They therefore ended up taking 'our drug' (long-acting methylphenidate) on five weekdays in the morning, followed by their 'drug' (cannabis) over the weekend. The above strategy, notwithstanding the risks involved, helped many youngsters to get back into mainstream education and helped achieve abstinence from cannabis in the long term.

Choice of medications to treat ADHD with comorbid substance misuse
There is a robust body of evidence from laboratory, clinical and neuroimaging studies to suggest that long-acting or controlled-release formulations are less likely to be misused than short-acting agents (Collins 2007). The abuse potential of oral methylphenidate is strongly influenced by its pharmacokinetic properties. The lower risk for misuse of extended-release formulations of methylphenidate is also related to the fact that its active components cannot be readily extracted (Wilens et al. 2006). The active compound contained in the osmotic controlled-release oral delivery system (OROS)-methylphenidate preparation is very difficult to extract by crushing, and the other long-acting stimulant formulations comprise long-acting beads that are not conducive to misuse by snorting, sniffing or injecting. These findings are consistent with a report on a group of adolescents with ADHD and substance misuse who were unable to achieve a high when attempting to inhale a preparation made from OROS methylphenidate (Jaffe 2002). However, despite their usefulness in producing high treatment adherence, whether treatment with extended-release stimulants is actually associated with a lower rate of misuse and/or reduced prevalence of substance misuse is a question that will require longer-term research.

Box 15.2: Clinicians can facilitate engagement in hard-to-reach young people in several ways

✓ Making use of the art of listening to young people – make them hear how they think!
✓ Appreciating the power imbalances in the therapeutic relationship
✓ Discovering the young person's strengths and resources
✓ Enhancing their motivation for change
✓ Instilling hope and rekindling their ability to dream about an alternative future

---

Box 15.3: Tips to use in a single-session MI-based assessment of substance use

✓ Assessment of substance misuse in the young is not rocket science! Clinicians working in CAMHS and Paediatrics already have the specialist skills to do the assessment.

✓ A safe space to talk and an empathic and non-judgmental stance from the clinician are crucial in encouraging young people to give details of their use of drugs and alcohol. Young people are more truthful than they are given credit for!

✓ The clinician facilitates rapport by expressing a genuine interest in and non-judgmental reactions to the young person's viewpoints and using language both familiar and similar to that of the clients.

✓ Collaboration works better than coercion: empathic listening and accurate reflection are crucial to facilitating change. If young people feel that they are truly understood and accepted by the clinician, they will be increasingly open to viewing the clinician as a valid consultant to their personal change process.

✓ Start off the assessment by asking about what they do for fun, what they get up to over the weekend – in a normative way. Ask for details of all drugs used, quantities, with whom, where, etc., including any risks endured.

✓ Establish the pattern of drug use and ascertain where they are in the developmental pathway/classification.

✓ You may choose to use one of the many strategies from motivational interviews (MI) to enhance their motivation to stop the use of drugs or to reduce harm.

✓ **Good things and Less Good things** (Box 15.4) is a useful strategy to use – especially in the early stages. It is useful for building rapport, and for understanding the context of substance use.

Box 15.4: The 'Good things and Less Good things' strategy for use in MI based assessment

✓ Use with clients who seem unconcerned, or when you are unsure about what they feel about their substance use. Resistance is minimised because you start with the positive things about the person's substance use.

✓ You talk about 'less good things' rather than 'concerns'. This allows the client to identify problem areas without feeling that these are being labelled as 'problematic'.

✓ Start off by asking the key question: 'What are some of the good things about your use of ....? (cannabis/alcohol)'. These usually emerge quickly. Summarise them if necessary. It may be helpful to write them down on one side of an A4 piece of paper.

✓ Then elicit the less good things about substances one by one, with the aim of finding out why this client thinks these are 'less good things'. Open questions are useful here, for example, 'How does this affect you?' or 'What don't you like about it?'. Write them down on the other side of the A4 sheet, so that you have a record of both on the same page.

✓ Summarise the good things and the less good things in 'you' language, as succinctly as possible, and leave the person time to react.

✓ For example: *'So using alcohol helps you relax... you enjoy doing this with friends, and it helps you when you are really fed up. On the other hand, you say you sometimes feel controlled by the stuff and that on Monday mornings you find it difficult to do anything at work'.*

✓ After the reflection, hand over the record of good things and less good things to the young person and ask them to reflect on it at home and add to/amend to it.

Lis-dexamfetamine dimesylate (LDX) is a promising new 'prodrug' formulation that could potentially reduce the risk of misuse of dexamphetamine by intranasal or intravenous routes. In its intact form, LDX is pharmacologically inactive. When taken orally, LDX is converted in the red blood cells by rate-limited enzymatic hydrolysis to L-lysine, a naturally occurring essential amino acid, and D-amphetamine. It has been proposed that this rate-limited conversion process may contribute to the extended duration of the effect that is seen throughout the day and a reduced 'drug liking' (Jasinski & Krishnan 2009), suggesting lower abuse potential. There is limited biotransformation of LDX when administered via parenteral routes. Double-blind crossover studies in adults with a history of stimulant misuse have suggested that the relative abuse potential of LDX was less than that for D-amphetamine (Jasinski et al. 2006). Early clinical experience is encouraging, but LDX has not yet been studied specifically in clinical populations with ADHD and comorbid substance misuse.

Atomoxetine, a selective norepinephrine reuptake inhibitor, has been reported to have little abuse potential, as evidenced by animal studies and small-scale studies in human volunteers (Heil et al. 2002; Wee & Woolverton 2004; Lile et al. 2006). Clinical experience is encouraging, although no randomised controlled trials have been carried out as yet to specifically assess the efficacy of atomoxetine in adolescents with ADHD and substance misuse. Meta-analytic studies and recent head-to-head studies have shown that the effect size of atomoxetine is somewhat lower compared to stimulants in the treatment of children and adults with ADHD without substance misuse (Faraone et al. 2006; Dittman et al. 2013). However, this issue is still arguable, and it has been suggested that the effect size of atomoxetine may become closer to that of the stimulants if a longer period of time (e.g. 12 weeks) is allowed and the person treated can tolerate the wait. However, in clinical practice, especially in young people with ADHD and comorbid substance misuse, we find that it is often difficult to achieve compliance with a longer period to full efficacy.

Guanfacine prolonged release is a new long-acting selective alpha 2-adrenoreceptor agonist, which has been shown to be effective in the treatment of ADHD, either alone or in combination with stimulants (Hervas et al. 2014) It has little abuse potential, although again, as yet, no clinical trials have been undertaken to attest the efficacy of guanfacine specifically in young people with people with ADHD and substance misuse.

The choice of a medication is dependent on the personal and family history of substance misuse, in particular the potential risk of misuse and diversion. In young people with non-chaotic substance abuse/dependence, and in the absence of significant family history of substance misuse, long-acting preparations of stimulant medications may be the preferred option, in view of their superior efficacy. However, if there is personal or family history of stimulant misuse and the substance misuse is chaotic, non-stimulants such as atomoxetine or guanfacine should be considered as the drugs of choice (Box 15.5).

Strategies to reduce diversion of stimulant medication

Patients at high risk of substance misuse or those with coexistent substance misuse should be monitored closely to ensure that optimal treatment efficacy is being achieved and that stimulants are not being misused or diverted (Box 15.6). It is crucial to inform young people and their parents about the potential for stimulants to be diverted for illicit use. Involving the family and/or other caregivers can substantially improve compliance with treatment, and reduce the likelihood of diversion of medication. Pointers such as drug-misusing relatives, being in a drug-misusing peer group, the combination of absence of effect with ongoing requests for prescriptions, and frequent mysterious 'loss' of prescriptions, should alert clinicians to the possibility of diversion and misuse of prescribed medication.

Box 15.5: Choice of medication to treat ADHD with coexisting substance misuse

Non-chaotic substance abuse/ dependence with alcohol, cannabis or tobacco and no personal or family history of stimulant misuse ⟶ Long-acting preparations of stimulant medications (e.g. Concerta XL, Medikinet XL or Equasym XL, or lisdexamphetamine)

Personal or family history of stimulant misuse and the substance misuse is chaotic; IV opiate use ⟶ Atomoxetine or guanfacine–prolonged release

---

Box 15.6: Recommended close monitoring of drug treatment to prevent diversion

Consider the following:

- ✓ More frequent visits (weekly or biweekly)
- ✓ Initial prescribing of smaller amounts of medication
- ✓ Parental supervision of medication
- ✓ Thorough record keeping of all prescription drugs
- ✓ The use of urine drug screens or other investigations to monitor illicit substance use
- ✓ Education of individuals with ADHD and their families regarding safe storage of the medication

> **Box 15.7:** Key practitioner messages
>
> ✓ Children with ADHD are at higher risk of developing substance misuse in adolescence and adulthood, and the risk is higher if there are comorbid conduct disorders and/or social adversity.
>
> ✓ There is a significant risk of development of nicotine abuse and dependence in people with ADHD, irrespective of the presence or absence of comorbid conduct disorder.
>
> ✓ The existing literature suggests that treatment of ADHD with medication does not increase the risk of the development of substance misuse.
>
> ✓ Misuse of stimulants employed for the treatment of ADHD is not uncommon, and stimulant medications are sometimes diverted and misused, either for subjective effects or for effects on performance.
>
> ✓ Integrated, multimodal treatment packages incorporating specific psychosocial and pharmacological treatment for substance misuse and other comorbidities such as conduct disorder should be provided along with optimal treatment of ADHD.
>
> ✓ Careful selection of agents for the treatment of patients with ADHD has the potential to limit drug diversion and misuse, particularly in high-risk groups such as those with a comorbid substance misuse or conduct disorder. Extended-release stimulants, non-stimulants or pro-drugs may be less likely to be misused or diverted.

Summary

- Substance misuse in adolescence is a major public health problem with substantial levels of morbidity and mortality. ADHD is a significant risk factor for the development of substance misuse through a number of complex causal pathways.

- Treatment of ADHD with medication is unlikely to increase the long-term risk of substance misuse. The risk of developing substance misuse is partly mediated by conduct problems (or the social adversity leading to them), and, therefore, psychosocial interventions should be offered as an integral part of the long-term treatment of ADHD, especially when there is psychiatric comorbidity.

- Young people with ADHD should be given specific information regarding the risk for substance misuse, and in particular the risk of development of nicotine dependence.

- Given the consistent findings of diversion and misuse of stimulants (either illicit use or for enhancing performance), clinicians, youth offending officers, substance misuse workers, teachers and other professionals should be made aware of the scope and context of the problem (Box 15.7).

- Specific programmes aimed at the prevention of substance misuse in children with ADHD and monitoring of prescription drug misuse and diversion should be developed with all stakeholders.

- Individuals identified with ADHD and comorbid substance misuse should be evaluated thoroughly for other complex needs and should be offered specific, evidence-based interventions to address both ADHD and substance misuse. The hope is that identification and optimal treatment of ADHD in children and adolescents may result in lower rates of substance misuse and diversion of stimulants, but further research is needed to establish whether this is in fact the case.

References

American Psychiatric Association (1994) *Diagnostic and statistical manual of mental disorders,* 4th edn. Washington, DC: American Psychiatric Association.

American Psychiatric Association (2013) *Diagnostic and statistical manual of mental disorders (DSM).* New York, NY: American Psychiatric Press.

Arias AJ, Gelernter J, Chan G et al. (2008) Correlates of co-occurring ADHD in drug-dependent subjects: Prevalence and features of substance dependence and psychiatric disorders. *Addictive Behav* 33(9): 1199–1207.

Barkley RA, Fischer M, Smallish L, Fletcher K (2004) Young adult follow-up of hyperactive children: Antisocial activities and drug use. *J Child Psychol Psychiatry* 45(2): 195–211.

Biederman J, Monuteaux MC, Mick E et al. (2006) Young adult outcome of attention deficit hyperactivity disorder: A controlled 10-year follow-up study. *Psychol Med* 36(2), 167–179.

Biederman J, Krishnan S, Zhang Y et al. (2007) Efficacy and tolerability of lisdexamfetamine dimesylate (NRP-104) in children with attention-deficit/hyperactivity disorder: A phase III, multicentre, randomized, double-blind, forced-dose, parallel-group study. *Clin Therapeut* 29: 450–463.

Biederman J, Monuteaux MC, Spencer T, Wilens TE, Macpherson HA, Faraone SV (2008) Stimulant therapy and risk for subsequent substance use disorders in male adults with ADHD: A naturalistic controlled 10-year follow-up study. *Am J Psychiatry* 65(5): 597–603.

Charach A, Yeung E, Climans T, Lillie E (2011) Childhood attention-deficit/hyperactivity disorder and future substance use disorders: Comparative meta-analyses. *J Am Acad Child Adolesc Psychiatry* 50: 9–21.

Collins S (2007) Abuse liability of medications used to treat attention-deficit/hyperactivity disorder. *Am J Addict* 16: 35–44.

Corless J, Mirza KAH, Steinglass P (2009) Family therapy for substance misuse: The maturation of a field. *J Fam Ther* 31: 109–114.

DiClemente CC, Schlundt D, Gemmell L (2004) Readiness and stages of change in addiction treatment. *Am J Addict* 13: 103–119.

Dittmann RW, Cardo E, Nagy P et al. (2013) Efficacy and safety of lisdexamfetamine dimesylate and atomoxetine in the treatment of attention-deficit/hyperactivity disorder: a head-to-head, randomized, double-blind, phase IIIb study. *CNS Drugs* 27: 1081–1092.

Faraone SV, Biederman J, Spencer TJ, Aleardi M (2006) Comparing the efficacy of medications for ADHD using meta-analysis. *Medscape Gen Med* 8: 4.

Faraone SV, Upadhyaya HP (2007) The effect of stimulant treatment for ADHD on later substance abuse and the potential for medication misuse, abuse, and diversion. *J Clin Psychiatry* 68(11): 28–35.

Geraghty O (2008) *An exploration of the black market availability and costs of licensed medicines in the North West* (MPharm dissertation). Liverpool: Liverpool John Moores University School of Pharmacy and Chemistry.

Gilvarry E (2000) Substance abuse in young people. *J Child Psychol Psychiatry* 41(1): 55–80.

Gilvarry E, McArdle P, Mirza KAH, Bevington D, Malcolm N (2012) *Practice standards for the assessment and treatment of children and young people with substance misuse* (publication no. CCQI 127). London: The Royal College of Psychiatrists.

Goldstein BI (2013) Do stimulants prevent substance use and misuse among youth with attention-deficit/hyperactivity disorder? The answer is still maybe. *J Am Acad Child Adolesc Psychiatry* 52(3): 225–227.

Greenhill LL, Pliszka S, Dulcan MK et al. (2002) Practice parameter for the use of stimulant medications in the treatment of children, adolescents, and adults. *J Am Acad Child Adolesc Psychiatry* 41(Suppl): 26S–49S.

Heil SH, Holmes HW, Bickela WK et al. (2002) Comparison of the subjective, physiological, and psychomotor effects of atomoxetine and methylphenidate in light drug users. *Drug Alcohol Depend* 67(2): 149–156.

Hervas A, Huss M, Johnson M et al. (2014) Efficacy and safety of extended-release guanfacine hydrochloride in children and adolescents with attention-deficit/hyperactivity disorder: A randomized, controlled, Phase III trial. *Eur Neuropsychopharmacol* 24(12): 1861–1872.

Hibell B et al. (2009) *The 2015 ESPAD Report: Substance use among students in 35 European countries.* Stockholm: The Swedish Council for Information on Alcohol and Other Drugs (CAN).

Home Office (2014) *Drug use: Findings from the 2012/13 Crime Survey for England and Wales.* Available at https://www.gov.uk/government/publications/drug-misuse-findings-from-the-2012-to-2013-csew.

Humphreys KL, Eng T, Lee SS (2013) Stimulant medication and substance use outcomes: A meta-analysis. *JAMA Psychiatry* 70: 740–749.

Huss M, Poustka F, Lehmkuhl G, Lehmkuhl U (2008) No increase in long-term risk for nicotine use disorders after treatment with methylphenidate in children with attention-deficit/hyperactivity disorder (ADHD): Evidence from a non-randomized retrospective study. *J Neural Transmission* 115(2): 335–339.

Jaffe SL (2002) Failed attempts at intranasal abuse of Concerta. *J Am Acad Child Adolesc Psychiatry* 41: 5.

Jasinski DR, Krishnan S (2009) Human pharmacology of intravenous lisdexamfetamine dimesylate: Abuse liability in adult stimulant abusers. *J Psychopharmacol* 23: 410–418.

Jasinski D, Krishnan S, Kehner G (2006) *Abuse liability of intravenous lisdexamfetamine* (LDX; NRP 104). Program and abstracts of the 2006 Annual Meeting of the Society for Developmental and Behavioral Pediatrics, 16–18 September, Philadelphia, PA.

Kandel DB (2002) *Stages and pathways of drug involvement: Examining the gateway hypothesis.* Cambridge, UK: Cambridge University Press, pp. 36–49.

Kollins SH, MacDonald EK, Rush CR (2001) Assessing the abuse potential of methyl phenidate in nonhuman and human subjects: A review. *Pharmacol Biochem Behav* 68: 611–627.

Lambert NM (2002) Stimulant treatment as a risk factor for nicotine use and substance abuse. In: Jensen PS, Cooper JR, editors. *Diagnosis and treatment of attention-deficit hyperactivity disorder: an evidence-based approach*, pp. 18-11–18-20. Kingston, NJ: Civic Research Institute.

Lee SS, Humphreys KL, Flory K, Liu R, Glass K (2011) Prospective association of childhood attention-deficit/hyperactivity disorder (ADHD) and substance use and abuse/dependence: A meta-analytic review. *Clin Psychol Rev* 31: 328–341.

Levin FR, Evans SM, Kleber HD (1998) Prevalence of adult attention-deficit hyperactivity disorder among cocaine abusers seeking treatment. *Drug Alcohol Dependence* 52(1): 15–25.

Lile JA, Stoops WW, Durell TM et al. (2006) Discriminative-stimulus, self-reported, performance, and cardiovascular effects of atomoxetine in methylphenidate-trained humans. *Exp Clin Psychopharmacol* 14(2): 136–147.

Mannuzza S, Klein RG, Truong NL et al. (2008) Age of methylphenidate treatment initiation in children with ADHD and later substance abuse: Prospective follow-up into adulthood. *Am J Psychiatry* 165: 604–609.

Marshall E, Mirza KAH (2007) Psychopharmacological treatment. In: Gilvarry E, McArdle P, editors. *Clinics in developmental medicine, alcohol, drugs and young people. Clinical approaches*, pp. 197–216. London: Mac Keith Press.

McCabe SE, Knight JR, Teter CJ, Weschler H (2005) Non medical use of prescription stimulants among US College students: Prevalence and correlates from a national survey. *Addiction* 99: 96–106.

McCambridge J, Strang J (2004) The efficacy of single-session motivational interviewing in reducing drug consumption and perceptions of drug-related risk and harm among young people: Results from a multi-site cluster randomised trial. *Addiction* 99: 39–52.

McCarthy S, Wilton L, Murray ML et al. (2012) The epidemiology of pharmacologically treated attention deficit hyperactivity disorder (ADHD) in children, adolescents and adults in UK primary care. *BMC Pediatrics* 12(78): 1–11.

Mirza KAH (2002) Adolescent substance use disorder In: Kutcher S, editor. *Practical child and adolescent psychopharmacology* (Cambridge monograph series), pp. 321–381. Cambridge: Cambridge University Press.

Mirza KAH, Buckstein O (2010) Assessment and treatment of young people with ADHD, disruptive behaviour disorder and co morbid substance use disorder. In: Kaminer Y, Winters K, editors. *Clinical manual of adolescent substance abuse treatment*, pp. 231–243. Washington, DC: American Psychiatric Publishing.

Mirza KAH, Sudesh RM, Mirza S (2011) Substance misuse in young people. In: Skuse D, Bruce H, Dowdney L, Mrazek D, editors. *Child psychology and psychiatry: Frameworks for practice*. London: John Wiley & Sons, pp. 201–209.

Mirza KAH, Sudesh R, Mirza S (2012) ADHD and substance misuse in young people: From cutting edge research to coal face reality of clinical practice. *Cutting Edge Psychiatry in Practice*, pp. 23–26.

Molina BSG, Flory K, Hinshaw SP et al. (2007) Delinquent behaviour and emerging substance use in MTA at 36 months: Prevalence, course, and treatment effects. *J Am Acad Child Adolesc Psychiatry* 46: 1–11.

Molina BSG, Hinshaw SP, Arnold LE et al. on behalf of the MTA (2013) Adolescent substance use in the multimodal treatment study of attention-deficit/hyperactivity disorder (ADHD) (MTA) as a function of childhood ADHD, random assignment to childhood treatments, and subsequent medication. *J Am Acad Child Adolesc Psychiatry* 52(3): 250–263.

NICE (2006) *Methylphenidate, atomoxetine and dexamphetamine for the treatment of attention deficit hyperactivity disorder in children and adolescents* (Technology Appraisal 98), London: NICE. Available at: www.nice.org.uk/TA98.

NICE (2008) *Attention deficit hyperactivity disorder: Diagnosis and management. NICE Clinical Guidelines* [CG72], https://www.nice.org.uk/guidance/cg72.

Nowinski J (1990) *Substance abuse in adolescents and young adults: A guide to treatment*, pp. 18–30. New York, NY: WW Norton & Company.

Parran TV, Jasinsky DR (1991) Intravenous methyphenidate abuse: Prototype for prescription drug abuse. *Arch Intern Med* 151: 781–783.

Riggs PD, Hall SK, Mikulich-Gilbertson SK, Lohman M, Kayser A (2004) A randomized controlled trial of pemoline for attention-deficit/hyperactivity disorder in substance-abusing adolescent. *J Am Acad Child Adolesc Psychiatry* 43(4): 420–429.

Riggs PD, Winhusen T, Davies RD et al. (2011) A randomized controlled trial of osmotic-release methylphenidate (OROS-MPH) for attention deficit hyperactivity disorder in adolescents with substance use disorders. *J Am Acad Child Adolesc Psychiatry* 50(9): 903–914.

Robbins TW (2002) ADHD and addiction. *Nat Med* 8(1): 24–25.

Robbins TW, Everitt BJ (2002) Limbic–striatal memory systems and drug addiction. *Neurobiol Learning Memory* 78(3): 625–636.

Schubiner H, Tzelepis A, Milberger S et al. (2000) Prevalence of attention-deficit/hyperactivity disorder and conduct disorder among substance abusers. *J Clin Psychiatry* 61(4): 244–251.

Steinhausen HC, Bisgaard C (2013) Substance use disorders in association with attention-deficit/hyperactivity disorder, co-morbid mental disorders, and medication in a nationwide sample. *Eur Neuropsychopharmacol* 24(2): 232–241.

Szobot CM, Rohde LA, Katz B et al. (2008) A randomised crossover clinical study showing that methylphenidate-SODAS improves attention-deficit/hyperactivity disorder symptoms in adolescents with substance use disorder. *Braz J Med Biol Res* 41(3): 250–257.

Taylor E (1986) The basis of drug treatment. In: *The overactive child*, pp. 196–198. Oxford: Blackwell Scientific.

Taylor E, Chadwick O, Heptinstall E et al. (1996) Hyperactivity and conduct problems as risk factors for adolescent development. *J Am Acad Child Adolesc Psychiatry* 35: 1213–1226.

Thurstone C, Riggs PD, Salomonsen-Sautel S, Mikulich-Gilbertson SK (2010) Randomized, controlled trial of atomoxetine for ADHD in adolescents with substance use disorder. *J Am Acad Child Adolesc Psychiatry* 49(6): 573–582.

Timimi S (2002) *Pathological child psychiatry and the medicalization of childhood*. Hove: Brunner; London: Routledge.

Volkow ND, Swanson JM (2003) Variables that affect the clinical use and abuse of methyl phenidate in the treatment of ADHD. *Am J Psychiatry* 160: 1909–1918.

Waldron HB, Kaminer Y (2004) On the learning curve: The emerging evidence supporting cognitive-behavioural therapies for adolescent substance abuse *Addiction* 99: 93–105.

Wee S, Woolverton WL (2004) Evaluation of the reinforcing effects of atomoxetine in monkeys: Comparison to methylphenidate and desipramine. *Drug Alcohol Depend* 75(3): 271–276.

WHO (1993) *The ICD-10 classification of mental and behavioural disorders: Clinical descriptions and diagnostic guidelines*. Geneva: World Health Organisation.

Wilens TE, Adler LA, Adams J et al. (2008) Misuse and diversion of stimulants prescribed for ADHD: A systematic review of the literature. *J Am Acad Child Adolesc Psychiatry* 47: 21–31.

Wilens TE, Bukstein O, Brams M et al. (2012) A controlled trial of extended release guanfacine and psychostimulants for ADHD. *J Am Acad Child Adolesc Psychiatry* 51(1): 74–85.

Wilens TE, Faraone SV, Biederman J, Gunawardene S (2003) Does stimulant therapy of attention-deficit/hyperactivity disorder beget later substance abuse? A meta-analytic review of the literature. *Paediatrics* 111(1): 179–185.

Wilens TE, Gignac M, Swezey A, Monuteaux MC, Biederman J (2006) Characteristics of adolescents and young adults with ADHD who divert or misuse their prescribed medications. *J Am Acad Child Adolesc Psychiatry* 45: 408–414.

Wilens TE, Martelon M, Joshi G et al. (2011) Does ADHD predict substance-use disorders? A 10-year follow-up study of young adults with ADHD. *J Am Acad Child Adolesc Psychiatry* 50(6): 543–553.

Williams RJ, Chang SY (2000) A comprehensive and comparative review of adolescent substance abuse treatment outcome. *Clin Psychol Sci Pract* 7: 138–166.

Woolfall K (2006) *Substance use among young people in Wirral, Merseyside.* Liverpool: Liverpool John Moores University.

Chapter 16

Transition to adult services in ADHD

Helen Crimlisk

Case scenario: Daniel

Daniel was diagnosed with ADHD aged 8. He also had some social skills difficulties but was a very intelligent child. His parents and school worked hard on managing his difficulties, and the use of medication also really helped. He did very well at GCSE. A levels were more of a struggle, but his school gave him detailed timelines for coursework and extra time to complete exams, so in the end things went well and he was accepted at a good university to study Information Technology. The University Special Needs Department knew a lot about ADHD and Kyle was well supported throughout his course. Medical follow-up was provided by the Student Health Services. On graduation, Dan was delighted to be offered a dream job working with a big company, which involved travelling overseas. Unfortunately he was then lost to follow-up until his paediatrician got a letter from him asking how he could get his medication in Italy as he had run out and needed it to manage his work.

Liam's childhood was spent yo-yoing between various members of his extended family and Local Authority Care. He missed a great deal of school and had attended at least eight schools by the age of 15. At 15 he was again in trouble with the police, and a lawyer who realised that he was a capable boy, despite all his difficulties, wondered about the diagnosis of ADHD. Daniel, however, continued to offend, and by the time it was agreed to assess him for ADHD he was over 16 and in an adult jail.

Ali is 24 years old. She went to see her GP about her 7-year-old son and the doctor referred him for assessment of possible ADHD. Ali struggled in school, but everyone just said she was lazy. She never got a real job. She got pregnant by mistake at 16 and now has two young children to care for. She tries to be a good mum but she finds it hard to organise everything and she often feels anxious and depressed.

Introduction: ADHD in adulthood

ADHD was traditionally seen as a disorder of children, diagnosed and treated by paediatricians and consultants in child and adolescent psychiatry. The general view was that children grew out of ADHD on reaching adulthood and, as such, the disorder was dealt with only by specialists in childhood disorders. This view probably relates to a perception that the main symptom of ADHD is that of hyperactivity. Although the psychopathology of ADHD does change over time, with a reduction in hyperactivity as children grow older, it is increasingly recognised that the other cardinal ADHD symptoms of inattention and impulsivity often do not decline to the same degree as motor symptoms and that adults with ADHD often experience an inner mental restlessness. The validity of the concept of ADHD in adults was examined and confirmed with publication of the NICE Guidelines on ADHD (NICE 2008), and there is increased recognition of ongoing symptoms and detrimental long-term outcomes in a significant proportion of young adults with ADHD (Klein et al. 2012).

A number of additional difficulties arising from this historical background make the concept of ADHD in adults harder to reconcile (Box 16.1). Commonly used diagnostic criteria still refer to symptoms relating to children, such as difficulty in the classroom, inability to complete homework, and so on. Retrospective history is harder to elicit reliably in adults: parents may not be available to describe childhood symptoms and young adults themselves usually under-recognise their past and present difficulties. Sometimes, coping strategies and the accumulation of positive skills or coping mechanisms may mask symptoms, even when the individual has ongoing needs.

In addition, comorbid disorders such as affective disorders, personality disorders and substance misuse may demand the attention of clinicians in adult services, resulting in

---

Box 16.1: Historical issues that impact on the concept of ADHD in adults

- ✓ Hyperactivity often declines leaving the less apparent symptoms
- ✓ Commonly used diagnostic criteria refer to childhood difficulties
- ✓ Retrospective history is harder to reliably elicit
- ✓ Coping strategies may mask symptoms
- ✓ Clinicians in adult services may pay more attention to the presenting disorder (co-morbid disorders such as affective disorders, personality disorders and substance misuse)
- ✓ Symptoms of ADHD may be of greater or lesser importance depending on the expectations and ambitions of the individual within their societal context

less attention being given to long-standing neurodevelopmental traits or disorders and more to the presenting disorder.

Finally, the range of socially acceptable behaviours, lifestyles and legitimate occupations in adulthood is wider than the more rigid expectations of the educational establishment in childhood. This means that symptoms of ADHD are of greater or lesser importance depending on the expectations and ambitions of the individual within their societal context.

In the UK, until the last decades of the twentieth century there were few adult services able to undertake diagnostic assessments in ADHD or take over the care of young adults with ADHD from children's services. This situation is changing rapidly, however, and service provision for adults with ADHD has developed, with leadership and training from The UK Adult ADHD Network (UKAAN; www.ukaan.org) and the Royal College of Psychiatry ADHD Network (www.rcpsych.ac.uk). ADHD in adults is now part of the curriculum for psychiatrists in training in the UK (Royal College of Psychiatrists 2010). The standards set out in the NICE Guidelines make it clear that diagnostic and ongoing treatment or follow-up should be provided in association with the commissioning structures in the UK (Kendall et al. 2008), and a variety of service models now exist for the diagnosis of ADHD in adults and for the follow-up of adults with ADHD on medication.

However, despite increased recognition of need, service provision in the UK and across the majority of the rest of Europe remains patchy, and it is often difficult for young people with ADHD and other neurodevelopmental disorders to make the transition into adult services successfully (Singh 2009; Hall et al. 2015). In the past, there was more flexibility for children's clinicians to treat young people into early (or even later) adulthood. However, although there are still some all-age services and there is increased interest in 0–25-year services (McGorry et al. 2013; Future in Mind 2015), service provision in the UK still usually means that at around the age of 18 years, arrangements need to be made with either adult mental health services or primary care to continue any necessary prescribing, other treatment and/or monitoring of both symptoms and potential side effects. In this chapter we will explore potential difficulties around transition and possible models of adult service provision, and consider strategies that may facilitate successful transition to appropriate adult provision in either primary or secondary care.

Disengagement from services or 'lost to follow-up'

Moving from Child and Adolescent Mental Health Services (CAMHS) or paediatrics to adult mental health services is beset by problems (Box 16.2). These include lack of information, poor provision, limited participation, limited engagement of the most vulnerable patients, varying adult eligibility thresholds and ring-fenced diagnostic limits of primary mental health services and specialist provision. There is also inconsistent

Box 16.2: Reasons why young people drop out of services at transition

✓ Young people actively choose to disengage

✓ Limited participation

✓ Limited engagement of the most vulnerable patients

✓ Varying adult eligibility thresholds

✓ Inconsistent or patchy support from all agencies

✓ Poor available provision

✓ Service is perceived as unwelcoming

✓ Parental input may wane or be rejected

✓ Rigidity of clinic timetabling and venue

✓ Limited flexibility for young people in terms of rearranging clinic appointments or re-engaging with services after a break

or patchy support, by both statutory and third-sector agencies who could provide psycho-education or self-management support (Pugh 2015). Accordingly, young people with ADHD may drop out of CAMHS or paediatrics, even before transition has been planned, or may not be offered follow-up because of poor attendance or failure to engage with adult provision.

There are a number of additional factors that sometimes contribute to this situation. For example, young people may struggle with the concept of ADHD or its treatment and actively choose to disengage (which is of course their right). They may struggle to cope with the rigidity of clinic timetabling or reject the service because of stigmatising associations that they perceive as unwelcoming. There is a tendency for paediatric and CAMHS clinics to be child focused rather than adolescent focused, which may be off-putting, but equally their reluctance to move to adult services may relate to the stigma associated with adult Community Mental Health Services or an atmosphere that is not experienced as 'young people friendly'. Parental input may wane at this point, or be rejected, and there may be limited flexibility for young people who are unable or choose not to attend in terms of rearranging clinic appointments or re-engaging with services after a break. Alarmingly frequently, young people may only re-engage at the point of crisis or after a negative event such as a psychological or social crisis or contact with the criminal justice system (Eme 2013).

Who should transition and to what?

A significant proportion of young people with ADHD in the UK have service needs at the point of discharge from children's services with an estimated 37% needing ongoing support from Adult Mental Health at the time of transition (Taylor et al. 2010).

Specialist nurses are common in children's services, and many young people (at least 36%) were felt likely to benefit from their input to support them at the time of transition and beyond. Such team members are, however, still unusual in adult services. The findings also suggested that general practitioners (GPs) could have a very positive role in management, with at least 50% of young people in the study being considered as 'well controlled' on medication. Adult mental health services in the UK are increasingly organised around the principal of providing 'care packages' (Department of Health 2013/2014), with people moving in and out of services for interventions as required. The concept of ADHD does not fit well into the structure of the current clustering arrangements. Primary care mental health services concentrate on treating 'common mental health conditions', which focus on depression and anxiety and do not currently have specialised skills around ADHD, although in view of the common comorbidity of depression and anxiety, it could be seen as appropriate that they develop further and that they could provide useful input to patients with ADHD.

There is disagreement about what proportion of young people with ADHD should transition to adult services. Some specialists suggest that all young people with ADHD should transition (Reale et al. 2014; Hall et al. 2015), while others believe that not all adults with ADHD will require adult mental health input (Marcer et al. 2008; Taylor et al. 2010; Young et al. 2011) as long as monitoring arrangements are in place in primary care, appropriate training and support is provided, and arrangements are available for review. For example, young people who are on stable medication regimens for ADHD may wish to continue this for many years into adulthood and are supported in doing this by NICE Guidelines (www.nice.org.uk/guidance/cg72). Such long-term monitoring is increasingly being passed on to primary care in a number of adult mental health disorders, although support, training and clear pathways for access back are required. In many cases where diagnoses have been undertaken by regional centres or privately, where there is no local provision or where young people have moved away from their homes (e.g. to university), GPs are left with little alternative to taking on monitoring and may also recognise that, when stable, monitoring is not complex. Shared care protocols in ADHD are common in children's services but less so in adult services, although there are a number of examples available on the Internet. In some areas, stable patients are discharged to primary care for monitoring under a shared care principle, with guidance and easy access to advice or reassessment.

When young people have not yet been stabilised on medication, experience side effects, have complex comorbidity or need further psycho-educational or psychological intervention for ADHD, they should be able to transition to appropriate adult services experienced in ADHD.

Box 16.3 considers the various possible options for service delivery models for adults with ADHD and the advantages and disadvantages of each.

Box 16.3: Service delivery models

Model	Advantages	Disadvantages
National/regional tertiary service	Centres of excellence Leaders in research and setting standards of service Expertise as a result of dedicated clinicians with significant experience	Geographically distant, with limited local knowledge Long-term follow-up not practical for many patients Difficult for some patients to access May attract an atypical client group because of the distances involved and the additional difficulties associated with obtaining funding for tertiary services
Neurodevelopmental disorders service	Experience in multidisciplinary assessment and diagnosis Dedicated staff with specialist experience Good links with neurology, paediatrics and intellectual disability services Good experience of liaison with education, vocational and occupational rehabilitation	Often have poor links with adult mental health services May not have skills to manage comorbid disorders
Age-defined local transitional service (e.g. for 15–25-year-olds)	Good links with CAMHS, paediatrics and intellectual disability services Early intervention at a critical point in transition between childhood and adulthood may have preventive value Extra support at a time when other areas of support may be lessening (e.g. education, family, children's services)	Problems inherent in a transitional service (bottleneck at age cut-off) Perceived as ageist
Local specialist ADHD team	Local expertise Easily accessible to service users May be better placed to negotiate local arrangements with the primary care trust (e.g. shared-care protocol)	Likely to be small May not see enough patients to develop expertise in more complex cases May not be truly multidisciplinary or integrated into teams

Box 16.3: Continued

Local (CMHT) embedded ADHD services	Local and easily accessible to service users	May not see enough patients to develop expertise in more complex cases
	Practical for a common disorder such as ADHD	Limited skills and experience – will need training
	Wide range of skills embedded within multidisciplinary team	Competition with other demands in CMHT
	Experience of managing comorbid problems	
	Good links with primary care	
Primary care-led service	Practical and local	Primary care physicians in the UK do not currently have the skills to diagnose or initiate treatment
	Best placed to oversee regular prescriptions and monitor patients	Most primary care physicians do not work within multidisciplinary teams that could assist management in more complex cases
	Use of shared care protocol can help primary care physicians decide how best to prescribe and monitor medication and when to seek help from secondary/ tertiary services	Will need access to more specialist advice regarding medication regimens, management of side–effects and discontinuation of medication
	Many general practices in the UK have access to psychological interventions that could help the common comorbidities of depression and anxiety	

Source: Reproduced, with permission, from Crimlisk (2011).

Reale and colleagues (2014) have set out an example of a decision tool that could help to inform the transition process and guide young people to the optimal service for their needs. Box 16.4 presents a simplified adaptation of this.

Transition to adult services

Of those who do make a transition, fewer than 5% experience adequate planning, continuity of care, good information transfer and joint working between teams (Kennedy 2010). Many transition service models are at an early stage of development or challenged by recent service reorganisations, and few robust effectiveness studies exist. The work of the TRACK (transition from CAMHS to adult mental health services) study (Singh et al. 2010) provided an understanding that good transition from child and adolescent mental health services to adult mental health services is rare and explored reasons for failure to

Box 16.4: Decision tool for the transition process

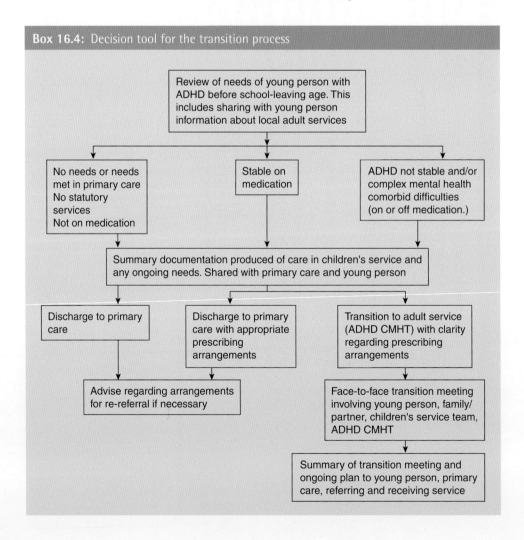

transfer. It called for further clinical outcomes-focused research on those who did and did not transfer. ADHD and other neurodevelopmental disorders were highlighted as an area of particular concern.

In England, the issue of transition is currently subject to unprecedented focus. A task force has been set up within NHS England to look into standards and implementation challenges of developing adolescent and transition pathways across the NHS (NHS England 2015a). The Joint Commissioning Panel Guidance for Commissioners of Mental Health Services for Young People in Transition sets out a series of principles and also references a number of case studies, including some on ADHD (JCPMH 2013). A model contract for commissioners has been written by NHS England (2015b) and NICE Guidelines (2015) on transition have recently been published and, while not making any firm recommendations about a model for transition, they do highlight a number of key factors (Box 16.5).

The concept of developmentally appropriate care

The concept of developmentally appropriate care – mapping service provision to the developmental level of the young person – is important at both ends of the age spectrum, demanding flexibility of approach from both adult and children's services (see Farre et al. 2015 for a discussion). Ambresin and colleagues (2013) have emphasised the features necessary for youth-friendly healthcare (summarised in Box 16.6) and these features provide a good checklist for considering the youth-friendliness of a service provision. It is important to

---

Box 16.5: NICE guidelines on transition: overarching principles

- ✓ Young people and carers involved in service design
- ✓ Use of person-centred approaches
- ✓ Health and Social Care to work in an integrated way
- ✓ Proactive identification and planning for young people with transition needs
- ✓ Sharing of safeguarding information
- ✓ Single named worker to coordinate transition
- ✓ Planning to be developmentally appropriate, not based on a rigid age threshold
- ✓ Transition planning to start from the age of 13 or 14
- ✓ Young people involved in transition through peer support, coaching, advocacy and/or mobile technology
- ✓ Focus on building independence – employment, education, inclusion, independent living, health and wellbeing
- ✓ Involvement of parents and carers
- ✓ Support before and after transition
- ✓ Training and development for staff
- ✓ Supporting infrastructure and senior organisational responsibility

note that the United Nations definition of 'youth' extends to 25 years, as it is clear that significant brain maturation is still occurring up to this point. Another factor that alters our perception of young people is that the nature of adolescence and young adulthood is changing. Young people are increasingly less financially independent of their parents. Transitions such as leaving home or starting work, which in previous generations commonly happened before the age of 20, are now increasingly uncommon until much later (Viner et al. 2012). This creates complexity with regards to our understanding of independence and adulthood, and arguably should prompt us to consider whether our binary model of service provision is the best we can do.

Preparation for transition and the role of peer support

There is increased emphasis on preparing young people to manage their own health and well-being. Transition projects in physical health, such as the Ready Steady Go Project (2015), emphasise transition as a process during which young people learn skills that will enable them to transition to the adult world safely. This project was devised for children with chronic physical disorders such as renal failure, diabetes and cystic fibrosis, and places emphasis on preparing for transition at an early point in the pathway (several years in advance of transition) and providing young people with tools to assist with transition by defining and monitoring their progress on a series of relevant competencies. Children and young adults move along a pathway annotated by a traffic light system moving towards transition date. There is an implicit assumption of flexibility of response, dependent on the needs and skills of the young person and close working between professionals on both sides of the transition boundary to ensure that the young people and their parents/carers are as informed as they need to be about the plan and their options. This approach seems relevant in the context of ADHD and comorbid conditions.

Box 16.6: Relevant indicators of adolescent-friendly services

✓ **Accessibility of health care:** location, affordability
✓ **Staff attitude:** respectful, supportive, honest, trustworthy, friendly
✓ **Communication:** clarity and provision of information, active listening, tone of communication
✓ **Medical competency:** technical skills (procedures)
✓ **Guideline–driven care:** confidentiality, autonomy, transition to adult healthcare services, comprehensive care
✓ **Age-appropriate environment:** flexibility of appointment times, separate physical space, teen-oriented health information, clean, waiting time, continuity of care, privacy
✓ **Involvement in healthcare**
✓ **Health outcomes:** pain management, quality of life

Source: Adapted from Ambresin et al. (2013).

Most guidelines also give weight to the importance of including the voice of the young person in service development. Excellent work looking into young people's views has been done by a number of third-sector agencies such as the Paul Hamlyn Foundation and Young Minds. Transition structures that incorporate service users in both service design and in providing peer support are advocated by many agencies. Young people may be more likely to listen to their peers and to be reassured by seeing young people who are successfully managing their condition and are coping with transition and the increasing demands of adulthood. There are some examples of ADHD-specific peer support development and transition clinics (SCIE 2011a,b), but there may also be advantages to concentrating on the generic needs of young people with mental health conditions in transition. The issues of symptom self-management, psycho-education, the necessity to explain their problems to others, social educational and employment problems and developing appropriate coping mechanisms to deal with stress and avoid relapse, may be more similar than any disorder-specific problems (SCIE 2011b).

Cultural and operational differences between adult and children's mental health services and specialist and generic services

Whereas children with ADHD may be supported by either CAMHS or paediatrics, adult services, where they exist, are likely to be either specialist ADHD services or generic Community Mental Health Teams (CMHTs). Both are likely to be led by adult psychiatrists, who may have variable multidisciplinary teams with nursing, psychology, occupational therapy, social care elements etc. A few have trained nurse prescribers, but this is not currently common in adult services. Most adult CMHTs in the UK operate a stepped-care model, with a primary mental health team that is commissioned around the treatment of common mental health conditions such as depression and anxiety, and a secondary mental health team based in a CMHT using an access and recovery model. The access team's function is rapid triage and assessment, along with consultation, advice and signposting functions. Recovery teams along with Crisis and Home treatment functions are intended for specific mental health intervention based on need and diagnosis using the Care and Clustering Package, which does not recognise/include ADHD or other neurodevelopmental disorders (Department of Health 2013/2014). CMHTs usually have a threshold based around severity, complexity and risk, which does not match well with CAMHS provision thresholds. The access and recovery models emphasise discharge to primary care if there are no specific interventions planned, and long-term follow-up is rare in the absence of major mental illness such as psychosis or significant risk. On the other hand, rapid access back into services in the event of relapse or crisis is better provided for in CMHTs, and the concept of consultation and advice to primary care is well established. As a more recently recognised disorder in adulthood, many adult psychiatrists and other mental health professionals and GPs will not have had specific training on ADHD, and they may need training to develop competencies in caring for this group of patients with confidence.

There are an increasing number of ADHD-specific adult services in the UK. Some of these are based around active research centres, while others have developed out of local initiatives and/or individual enthusiasm or expertise. These services have the advantage of specific expertise and a focus on ADHD (and often other neurodevelopmental disorders), and encourage the recruitment of patients into research trials. For individuals who can get to them, they provide a valuable service. However, non-attendance and disengagement is common in ADHD, and there may be difficulties for young people, particularly those who are socially disadvantaged, in travelling to specialist centres. These features mean that specialist services, which tend to be less close to patients' homes, less flexible in approach and less well connected to generic mental health teams, also have disadvantages. The breadth of mental and social care service provision that may be necessary to help patients with ADHD is probably better served by local service providers supported by specialist centres of excellence as required (see Box 16.3 and also Crimlisk 2011 for further discussion).

Teams working together over the transition period

The current focus on transition in England is welcomed as a driver to encourage children's and adult services to work together to ensure that the transition process for young people with ADHD is an opportunity for a constructive process. As well as minimising the potential disruption of any change in professionals or structural organisation, there should be a focus on developing the skills necessary for the wider transition that the young person is undergoing into adulthood. This will include self-management techniques, knowledge around accessing services, and developing the confidence to seek out additional sources of help. To facilitate a successful transition, a range of structural features are likely to help. A familiar setting for an initial meeting will increase attendance, and the involvement of a key person whom the young person knows is likely to ensure that the new team or professional benefits from trust developed over years. The young person should be actively involved in the process and they and relevant family/friends should have the opportunity to ask questions, receive written information and be given clear instructions as to how to obtain their medication, whom to call in an emergency and what to expect from follow-up. A period of joint working may be valuable, and a comprehensive case summary should be prepared. The outcome of the meeting should be clearly documented and shared with the young person and the GP (Box 16.4).

The development of a service model for adults with ADHD in Sheffield is described in Crimlisk (2011). As a part of this model, a peer-supported transition group has been developed for young adults. The module components (adapted from Young & Bramham 2007) are shown in Box 16.7. There is a useful leaflet about adult ADHD on the Royal College of Psychiatry website (http://www.rcpsych.ac.uk/healthadvice/problemsdisorders/adhdinadults.aspx), which can be printed off free and given to young people with ADHD and their partners or family. It is also useful to share self-help tips for living with ADHD with young adults and those with whom they share their lives (Box 16.8, reproduced with permission from The Royal College of Psychiatrists).

Box 16.7: Elements within 'Transition Group Curriculum relevant to ADHD'

✓ Managing anger
✓ Time management and prioritising
✓ Regulating activity levels
✓ Self esteem and negative thoughts
✓ Planning and impulsivity
✓ Use of substances: medication and others
✓ Memory and problem solving
✓ Learning to learn effectively
✓ Choosing and keeping friends
✓ Keeping out of trouble
✓ Scary situations: managing anxiety

Source: Amended, with permission, from Crimlisk (2011).

Box 16.8: Fifteen tips to help you manage your ADHD

✓ **Tell people** : But don't use the diagnosis as an 'excuse'
✓ **Ask for help from your friends and family** : But say exactly what you need
✓ **Get feedback about how you affect others** : And ask for feedback about when you do things well
✓ **Use structure and prioritise** : Make lists and notes, use colour coding and reminders, write down plans, break down big goals into smaller, manageable tasks
✓ **Reward yourself when things go well** : Or don't go too badly!
✓ **Respond to boring tasks quickly** : 'OHIO' = only handle it once
✓ **Accept that some things are just difficult** : So it doesn't get you down
✓ **Plan difficult meetings or conversations** : Anticipate problems
✓ **Find ways to help yourself concentrate** : Background music, silence, something to 'fiddle with' in your hands
✓ **Have 'blow-out time' or 'time outs'** : Gym, dancing, running
✓ **Don't beat yourself up** : (Or your parents or partner!)
✓ **Join a support group** : Or start one!
✓ **Learn to tolerate your moods** : (Without panicking or catastrophising) NOT 'I'm hopeless' or 'I never manage to...'
✓ **Find friends who are good for you** : And spend time with them
✓ **Be proud of yourself** : Yes really...you're trying to make things better!

Source: Adapted from '50 Tips for ADHD by Ed Hallowell', http://www.drhallowell.com/adult-adhd-50-tips-of-management/.

Summary

- As ADHD is increasingly recognised as a common condition in adulthood, with significant long-term academic, social and psychological consequences, it will be necessary to consider alternative service delivery models for this population.

- Clearly, the period around adolescence and early adulthood is a key time, when the consequences of behaviours mediated by ADHD could have a significant negative impact on a young person's life (e.g. educational underachievement, low self-esteem, risky behaviour, substance misuse and criminal behaviour). Given this critical time, a service design that does not involve transition in the middle of this would be sensible.

- The move towards 0–25 years services would go some way to ameliorating the negative consequences of transition and focusing on early interventions in early adult life to maximise potential. For some patients and professionals this will still be seen as inadequate, as ADHD is seen as a long-term or indeed life-long condition. It seems unlikely, however, that lifelong single disorder service provision will be feasible and it goes against the current drivers in managing long-term conditions (Turgay et al. 2012).

- It may be that technology offers alternative innovative service models that may be useful.

- Whatever the model, transition between teams is likely to continue to be an issue and the principles discussed in this chapter and the references to evidence them will continue to be relevant and valuable, regardless of the organisational structures in place in the future (Myers et al. 2015).

References

Ambresin A, Bennett K, Patton G, Sanci L, Sawyer S (2013) Assessment of youth-friendly health care: A systematic review of indicators drawn from young people's perspectives. *J Adolesc Health* 52: 670–681, doi:10.1016/j.jadohealth.2012.12.014.

Crimlisk H (2011) Developing integrated mental health services for adults with ADHD. *Adv Psychiatr Treatment* 17(6): 461–469, doi:10.1192/apt.bp.109.00692.

Department of Health (2013/2014) *Mental health clustering and payment by results*; available at https://www.gov.uk/government/publications/mental-health-payment-by-results-arrangements-for-2013-14.

Eme R (2013) Attention-deficit/hyperactivity disorder and criminal behavior. *Int J Sociol* 1(2): 29–36.

Farre A, Wood V, Rapley JR, Parr JR, Reape D, McDonagh JE (2015) Developmentally appropriate healthcare for young people: A scoping study. *Arch Dis Child* 100(2): 144–151, doi:10.1136/archdischild-2014-306749.

Future in Mind (2015) *Promoting, protecting and improving our children and young people's mental health and wellbeing*; available at https://www.gov.uk/government/publications/improving-mental-health-services-for-young-people.

Hall CL, Newell K, Taylor J, Sayal K, Hollis C (2015) Services for young people with attention deficit/hyperactivity disorder transitioning from child to adult mental health services: A national survey of mental health trusts in England. *J Psychopharmacol* 29(1): 39–42.

JCPMH (2013) Available at www.jcpmh.info/good-services/young-people-in-transition.

Kendall T, Taylor E, Perez A, Taylor C and the Guideline Development Group (2008) Diagnosis and management of attention-deficit/hyperactivity disorder in children, young people, and adults: Summary of NICE guidance. *Br Med J* 337: a1239, doi:10.1136/bmj.a1239.

Kennedy I (2010) *Getting it right for children and young people – Overcoming cultural barriers in the NHS so as to meet their needs.* London: Department of Health.

Klein RG, Mannuzza S, Olazagasti MA et al. (2012) Clinical and functional outcome of childhood attention deficit/hyperactivity disorder 33 years later. *Arch Gen Psychiatry* 69(12): 1295–1303, doi:10.1001/archgenpsychiatry.2012.271.

Marcer H, Finlay F, Baverstock A (2008) ADHD and transition to adult services – The experience of community paediatricians. *Child Care Health Dev* 34(5): 564–566, doi:10.1111/j.1365-2214.2008.00857.x.

McGorry P, Bates T, Birchwood M (2013) Designing youth mental health services for the 21st century: Examples from Australia, Ireland and the UK. *Br J Psychiatry* 202(s54): s30–s35, doi:10.1192/bjp.bp.112.119214.

Myers K, Vander Stoep A, Zhou C, McCarty CA, Katon W (2015) Effectiveness of a telehealth service delivery model for treating attention-deficit/hyperactivity disorder: A community-based randomized controlled trial. *J Am Acad Child Adolesc Psychiatry* 54(4): 263–274, doi:10.1016/j.jaac.2015.01.009.

NHS England (2015a) *Improving transition for children and young people*; available at https://www.england.nhs.uk/tag/transition/.

NHS England (2015b) *NHS standard contract model transfer of and discharge from care protocol for young people with mental health problems in transition from CAMHS*; available at https://www.england.nhs.uk/wp-content/uploads/2015/01/mod-camhs-transt-prot.pdf.

NHS England Joint Commissioning Panel for Mental Health (2013) *Young people in transition*; available at http://www.jcpmh.info/good-services/young-people-in-transition/.

NICE (2008) *Attention deficit hyperactivity disorder: Diagnosis and management. NICE Clinical Guidelines* [CG72], https://www.nice.org.uk/guidance/cg72.

NICE (2015) *Transition from children's to adults' services: draft guideline consultation*; available at https://www.nice.org.uk/guidance/ng43.

Paul Hamlyn Foundation; available at http://www.phf.org.uk.

Pugh K (2015) *Model specification for transitions from child and adolescent mental health services.* London: NHS England.

Ready Steady Go (2015) *Transition to adult care: Ready steady go*; available at https://www.jfhc.co.uk/saphna/ready_steady_go.aspx.

Reale L, Frassica S, Gollner A, Bonati M (2015) Transition to adult mental health services for young people with ADHD. *Postgrad Med* 127(7): 671–676.

Royal College of Psychiatrists (2010) *Royal College of Psychiatry core curriculum*; available at http://www.rcpsych.ac.uk/pdf/CORE_CURRICULUM_2010_Mar_2012_update.pdf.

Singh SP (2009) Transition of care from child to adult mental health services: The great divide. *Curr Opin Psychiatry* 22(4): 386–390, doi:10.1097/YCO.0b013e32832c9221.

Singh SP, Paul M, Ford T et al. (2010) Process, outcome and experience of transtion from child to adult mental healthcare: Multiperspective study. *Br J Psychiatry* 197(4): 305–312, doi:10.1192/bjp.bp.109.075135.

Social Care Institute of Excellence (2011a) *Transition case studies*; see http://staging.scie-socialcareonline.org.uk/case-study-sheffield-adhd-transitions/r/a11900000017rwj1ay.

Social Care Institute of Excellence (2011b) Transition clinics and transition groups; available at http://www.scie.org.uk/socialcaretv/topic.asp?t=mentalhealthtransitions.

Taylor N, Fauset A, Harpin V (2010) Young adults with ADHD: An analysis of their service needs on transfer to adult services. *Arch Dis Child* 95(7): 513–517, doi:10.1136/adc.2009.164384.

Turgay A, Goodman DW, Asherson P et al. (2012) Lifespan persistence of ADHD: The life transition model and its application. *J Clin Psychiatry* 73(2): 192–201, doi:10.4088/JCP.10m06628.

UKAAN; available at http://www.ukaan.org.

Viner RM, Ozer EM, Denny S et al. (2012) Adolescence and the social determinants of health. *Lancet* 379(9826): 1641–1652, doi:10.1016/S0140-6736(12)60149-4.

Young Minds; available at http://www.youngminds.org.uk/.

Young S, Bramham J (2007) *Cognitive behavioural therapy for ADHD in adults and adolescents: A psychological guide to practice*, 2nd edn. London: Wiley.

Young S, Murphy CM, Coghill D (2011) Avoiding the 'twilight zone': Recommendations for the transition of services from adolescence to adulthood for young people with ADHD. *BMC Psychiatry* 11: 174.

Appendices

Appendix 1   Useful websites for you or the family you support

- https://www.nice.org.uk/guidance/cg72/ifp/chapter/information-for-parents-of-children-with-adhd
- http://www.youngminds.org.uk/for_parents/worried_about_your_child/adhd_children
- www.adhd-institute.com (information for professionals sponsored by Shire Pharmaceuticals)
- www.addiss.co.uk
- www.adhdandjustice.co.uk

Parent resources and conferences:

- https://www.nice.org.uk/guidance/cg72
- http://www.ukadhd.com
- The UK ADHD Partnership
- www.cafamily.org.uk (general information, e.g. around Education Health Care Plans or Disability Living Allowance and specific information about ADHD for parents and professionals)
- http://caddra.ca (includes information for health professionals, teachers, parents and young people)
- www.chadd.org (CHADD – The National Resource on ADHD: parent information and conferences)
- www.ukaan.org (UKAAN is a professional body that aims to support practitioners in rolling out NICE Clinical Guideline 72 and establish clinical services for adults in the UK)
- http://www.adhdvoices.com (gives insight into how children and young people feel about their ADHD and the treatment they receive)

Appendix 2a Blood pressure (BP) levels for boys by age and height centile*

Age (years)	BP centile ↓	Systolic BP (mmHg) ← Centile of height →							Diastolic BP (mmHg) ← Centile of height →						
		5th	10th	25th	50th	75th	90th	95th	5th	10th	25th	50th	75th	90th	95th
1	50th	80	81	83	85	87	88	89	34	35	36	37	38	39	39
	90th	94	95	97	99	100	102	103	49	50	51	52	53	53	54
	95th	98	99	101	103	104	106	106	54	54	55	56	57	58	58
	99th	105	106	108	110	112	113	114	61	62	63	64	65	66	66
2	50th	84	85	87	88	90	92	92	39	40	41	42	43	44	44
	90th	97	99	100	102	104	105	106	54	55	56	57	58	58	59
	95th	101	102	104	106	108	109	110	59	59	60	61	62	63	63
	99th	109	110	111	113	115	117	117	66	67	68	69	70	71	71
3	50th	86	87	89	91	93	94	95	44	44	45	46	47	48	48
	90th	100	101	103	105	107	108	109	59	59	60	61	62	63	63
	95th	104	105	107	109	110	112	113	63	63	64	65	66	67	67
	99th	111	112	114	116	118	119	120	71	71	72	73	74	75	75
4	50th	88	89	91	93	95	96	97	47	48	49	50	51	51	52
	90th	102	103	105	107	109	110	111	62	63	64	65	66	66	67
	95th	106	107	109	111	112	114	115	66	67	68	69	70	71	71
	99th	113	114	116	118	120	121	122	74	75	76	77	78	78	79
5	50th	90	91	93	95	96	98	98	50	51	52	53	54	55	55
	90th	104	105	106	108	110	111	112	65	66	67	68	69	69	70
	95th	108	109	110	112	114	115	116	69	70	71	72	73	74	74
	99th	115	116	118	120	121	123	123	77	78	79	80	81	81	82
6	50th	91	92	94	96	98	99	100	53	53	54	55	56	57	57
	90th	105	106	108	110	111	113	113	68	68	69	70	71	72	72
	95th	109	110	112	114	115	117	117	72	72	73	74	75	76	76
	99th	116	117	119	121	123	124	125	80	80	81	82	83	84	84
7	50th	95	94	95	97	99	100	101	55	55	56	57	58	59	59
	90th	106	107	109	111	113	114	115	70	70	71	72	73	74	74
	95th	110	111	113	115	117	118	119	74	74	75	76	77	78	78
	99th	117	118	120	122	124	125	126	82	82	83	84	85	86	86
8	50th	94	95	97	99	100	102	102	56	57	58	59	60	60	61
	90th	107	109	110	112	114	115	116	71	72	72	73	74	75	76
	95th	111	112	114	116	118	119	120	75	76	77	78	79	79	80
	99th	119	120	122	123	125	127	127	83	84	85	86	87	87	88
9	50th	95	96	98	100	102	103	104	57	58	59	60	61	61	62
	90th	109	110	112	114	115	117	118	72	73	74	75	76	76	77
	95th	113	114	116	118	119	121	121	76	77	78	79	80	81	81
	99th	120	121	123	125	127	128	129	84	85	86	87	88	88	89
10	50th	97	98	100	102	103	105	106	58	59	60	61	61	62	63
	90th	111	112	114	115	117	119	119	73	73	74	75	76	77	78

Appendix 2a (Continued)

Age (years)	BP centile ↓	Systolic BP (mmHg) ← Centile of height →							Diastolic BP (mmHg) ← Centile of height →						
		5th	10th	25th	50th	75th	90th	95th	5th	10th	25th	50th	75th	90th	95th
	95th	115	116	117	119	121	122	123	77	78	79	80	81	81	82
	99th	122	123	125	127	128	130	130	85	86	86	88	88	89	90
11	50th	99	100	102	104	105	107	107	59	59	60	61	62	63	63
	90th	113	114	115	117	119	120	121	74	74	75	76	77	78	78
	95th	117	118	119	121	123	124	125	78	78	79	80	81	82	82
	99th	124	125	127	129	130	132	132	86	86	87	88	89	90	90
12	50th	101	102	104	106	108	109	110	59	60	61	62	63	63	64
	90th	115	116	118	120	121	123	123	74	75	75	76	77	78	79
	95th	119	120	122	123	125	127	127	78	79	80	81	82	82	83
	99th	126	127	129	131	133	134	135	86	87	88	89	90	90	91
13	50th	104	105	106	108	110	111	112	60	60	61	62	63	64	64
	90th	117	118	120	122	124	125	126	75	75	76	77	78	79	79
	95th	121	122	124	126	128	129	130	79	79	80	81	82	83	83
	99th	128	130	131	133	135	136	137	87	87	88	89	90	91	91
14	50th	106	107	109	111	113	114	115	60	61	62	63	64	65	65
	90th	120	121	123	125	126	128	128	75	76	77	78	79	79	80
	95th	124	125	127	128	130	132	132	80	80	81	82	83	84	84
	99th	131	132	134	136	138	139	140	87	88	89	90	91	92	92
15	50th	109	110	112	113	115	117	117	61	62	63	64	65	66	66
	90th	122	124	125	127	129	130	131	76	77	78	79	80	80	81
	95th	126	127	129	131	133	134	135	81	81	82	83	84	85	85
	99th	134	135	136	138	140	142	142	88	89	90	91	92	93	93
16	50th	111	112	114	116	118	119	120	63	63	64	65	66	67	67
	90th	125	126	128	130	131	133	134	78	78	79	80	81	82	82
	95th	129	130	132	134	135	137	137	82	83	83	84	85	86	87
	99th	136	137	139	141	143	144	145	90	90	91	92	93	94	94
17	50th	114	115	116	118	120	121	122	65	66	66	67	68	69	70
	90th	127	128	130	132	134	135	136	80	80	81	82	83	84	84
	95th	131	132	134	136	138	139	140	84	85	86	87	87	88	89
	99th	139	140	141	143	145	146	147	92	93	93	94	95	96	97

*The 90th centile is 1.28 SD, 95th centile is 1.645 SD and the 99th centile is 2.326 SD over the mean. For research purposes, the standard deviations in appendix table B–1 allow one to compute BP Z-scores and centiles for boys with height centiles given in table 3 (i.e. the 5th, 10th, 25th, 50th, 75th, 90th and 95th centiles). These height centiles must be converted to height Z-scores given by (5%=−1.645; 10%=−1.28; 25%=−0.68; 50%=0; 75%=0.68; 90%=1.28; 95%=1.645) and then computed according to the methodology in steps 2–4 described in Appendix B. For children with height centiles other than these, follow steps 1–4 as described in Appendix B.

Appendix 2b   Blood pressure (BP) levels for girls by age and height centile*

Age (years)	BP centile ↓	Systolic BP (mmHg) ← Centile of height →							Diastolic BP (mmHg) ← Centile of height →						
		5th	10th	25th	50th	75th	90th	95th	5th	10th	25th	50th	75th	90th	95th
1	50th	83	84	85	86	88	89	90	38	39	39	40	41	41	42
	90th	97	97	98	100	101	102	103	52	53	53	54	55	55	56
	95th	100	101	102	104	105	106	107	56	57	57	58	59	59	60
	99th	108	108	109	111	112	113	114	64	64	65	65	66	67	67
2	50th	85	85	87	88	89	91	91	43	44	44	45	46	46	47
	90th	98	99	100	101	103	104	105	57	58	58	59	60	61	61
	95th	102	103	104	105	107	108	109	61	62	62	63	64	65	65
	99th	109	110	111	112	114	115	116	69	69	70	70	71	72	72
3	50th	86	87	88	89	91	92	93	47	48	48	49	50	50	51
	90th	100	100	102	103	104	106	106	61	62	62	63	64	64	65
	95th	104	104	105	107	108	109	110	65	66	66	67	68	68	69
	99th	111	111	113	114	115	116	117	73	73	74	74	75	76	76
4	50th	88	88	90	91	92	94	94	50	50	51	52	52	53	54
	90th	101	102	103	104	106	107	108	64	64	65	66	67	67	68
	95th	105	106	107	108	110	111	112	68	68	69	70	71	71	72
	99th	112	113	114	115	117	118	119	76	76	76	77	78	79	79
5	50th	89	90	91	93	94	95	96	52	53	53	54	55	55	56
	90th	103	103	105	106	107	109	109	66	67	67	68	69	69	70
	95th	107	107	108	110	111	112	113	70	71	71	72	73	73	74
	99th	114	114	116	117	118	120	120	78	78	79	79	80	81	81
6	50th	91	92	93	94	96	97	98	54	54	55	56	56	57	58
	90th	104	105	106	108	109	110	111	68	68	69	70	70	71	72
	95th	108	109	110	111	113	114	115	72	72	73	74	74	75	76
	99th	115	116	117	119	120	121	122	80	80	80	81	82	83	83
7	50th	93	93	95	96	97	99	99	55	56	56	57	58	58	59
	90th	106	107	108	109	111	112	113	69	70	70	71	72	72	73
	95th	110	111	112	113	115	116	116	73	74	74	75	76	76	77
	99th	117	118	119	120	122	123	124	81	81	82	82	83	84	84
8	50th	95	95	96	98	99	100	101	57	57	57	58	59	60	60
	90th	108	109	110	111	113	114	114	71	71	71	72	73	74	74
	95th	112	112	114	115	116	118	118	75	75	75	76	77	78	78
	99th	119	120	121	122	123	125	125	82	82	83	83	84	85	86
9	50th	96	97	98	100	101	102	103	58	58	58	59	60	61	61
	90th	110	110	112	113	114	116	116	72	72	72	73	74	75	75
	95th	114	114	115	117	118	119	120	76	76	76	77	78	79	79
	99th	121	121	123	124	125	127	127	83	83	84	84	85	86	87
10	50th	98	99	100	102	103	104	105	59	59	59	60	61	62	62
	90th	112	112	114	115	116	118	118	73	73	73	74	75	76	76

Appendix 2b (Continued)

Age (years)	BP centile ↓	Systolic BP (mmHg) ← Centile of height →							Diastolic BP (mmHg) ← Centile of height →						
		5th	10th	25th	50th	75th	90th	95th	5th	10th	25th	50th	75th	90th	95th
	95th	116	116	117	119	120	121	122	77	77	77	78	79	80	80
	99th	123	123	125	126	127	129	129	84	84	85	86	86	87	88
11	50th	100	101	102	103	105	106	107	60	60	60	61	62	63	63
	90th	114	114	116	117	118	119	120	74	74	74	75	76	77	77
	95th	118	118	119	121	122	123	124	78	78	78	79	80	81	81
	99th	125	125	126	128	129	130	131	85	85	86	87	87	88	89
12	50th	102	103	104	105	107	108	109	61	61	61	62	63	64	64
	90th	116	116	117	119	120	121	122	75	75	75	76	77	78	78
	95th	119	120	121	123	124	125	126	79	79	79	80	81	82	82
	99th	127	127	128	130	131	132	133	86	86	87	88	88	89	90
13	50th	104	105	106	107	109	110	110	62	62	62	63	64	65	65
	90th	117	118	119	121	122	123	124	76	76	76	77	78	79	79
	95th	121	122	123	124	126	127	128	80	80	80	81	82	83	83
	99th	128	129	130	132	133	134	135	87	87	88	89	89	90	91
14	50th	106	106	107	109	110	111	112	63	63	63	64	65	66	66
	90th	119	120	121	122	124	125	125	77	77	77	78	79	80	80
	95th	123	123	125	126	127	129	129	81	81	81	82	83	84	84
	99th	130	131	132	133	135	136	136	88	88	89	90	90	91	92
15	50th	107	108	109	110	111	113	113	64	64	64	65	66	67	67
	90th	120	121	122	123	125	126	127	78	78	78	79	80	81	81
	95th	124	125	126	127	129	130	131	82	82	82	83	84	85	85
	99th	131	132	133	134	136	137	138	89	89	90	91	91	92	93
16	50th	108	108	110	111	112	114	114	64	64	65	66	66	67	68
	90th	121	122	123	124	126	127	128	78	78	79	80	81	81	82
	95th	125	126	127	128	130	131	132	82	82	83	84	85	85	86
	99th	132	133	134	135	137	138	139	90	90	90	91	92	93	93
17	50th	108	109	110	111	113	114	115	64	65	65	66	67	67	68
	90th	122	122	123	125	126	127	128	78	79	79	80	81	81	82
	95th	125	126	127	129	130	131	132	82	83	83	84	85	85	86
	99th	133	133	134	136	137	138	139	90	90	91	91	92	93	93

*The 90th centile is 1.28 SD, 95th centile is 1.645 SD and the 99th centile is 2.326 SD over the mean. For research purposes, the standard deviations in appendix table B–1 allow one to compute BP Z-scores and centiles for girls with height centiles given in table 4 (i.e. the 5th, 10th, 25th, 50th, 75th, 90th and 95th centiles). These height centiles must be converted to height Z-scores given by (5%=−1.645; 10%=−1.28; 25%=−0.68; 50%=0; 75%=0.68; 90%=1.28; 95% = 1.645) and then computed according to the methodology in steps 2–4 described in Appendix B. For children with height centiles other than these, follow steps 1–4 as described in Appendix B.

Appendix 2c   Recommended dimensions for blood pressure cuff bladders

Age range	Width (cm)	Length (cm)	Maximum arm circumference (cm)*
Newborn	4	8	10
Infant	6	12	15
Child	9	18	22
Small adult	10	24	26
Adult	13	30	34
Large adult	16	38	44
Thigh	20	42	52

* Calculated so that the largest arm would still allow bladder to encircle arm by at least 80%.

Appendix 3   Normal ranges of resting heart rate in beats per minute (bpm)

Age in years:

- ✓ 2–5: 95–140 bpm
- ✓ 5–12: 80–120 bpm
- ✓ >12: 60–100 bpm

Tachyarrhythmia needs exclusion if a school-aged child has a heart rate >160 beats/minute

Appendix 4a   Care pathway: Management of ADHD in preschool children

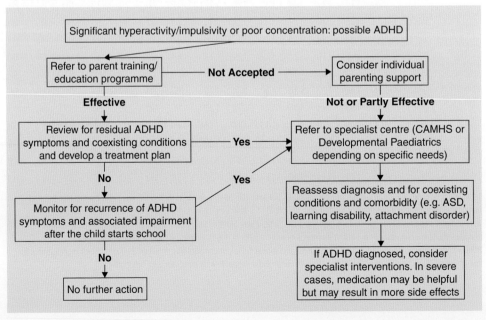

Appendix 4b Care pathway: Management of ADHD in school age children and young people

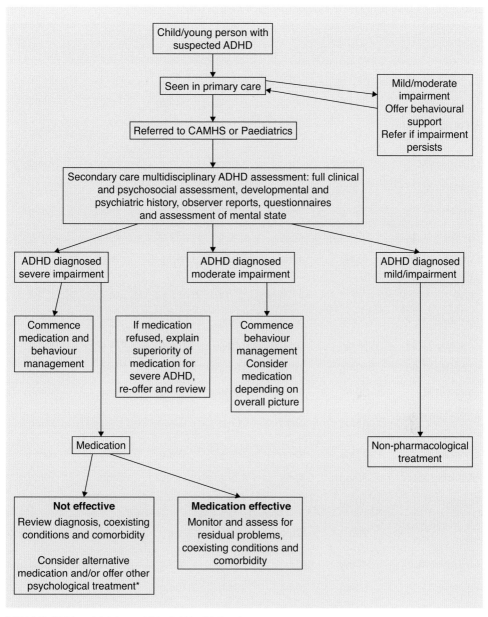

* CAMHS, Child and Adolescent Mental Health Services

Appendix 5a A comparison of extended release methylphenidate preparations showing the amount of methylphenidate release during each time period

Product	Stated content	0–4h	4–8h	8–12h	>12h	Total release
Concerta XL 18	18mg	2mg	5mg	4mg	4mg	15mg
Equasym XL	10mg	3mg	4mg	2mg	1mg	10mg
Methylphenidate plain	5mg	3mg	2mg	–	–	5mg
Medikinet XL	10mg	3mg	4mg	2mg	1mg	10mg
Concerta XL 27	27mg	4mg	7mg	7mg	5mg	22.5mg
Concerta XL 36	36mg	5mg	9mg	9mg	7mg	30mg
Equasym XL	20mg	6mg	7mg	4mg	2mg	20mg
Concerta XL 45	45mg	6mg	11mg	11mg	9mg	37.5mg
Methylphenidate plain	10mg	6mg	4mg	–	–	10mg
Medikinet XL	20mg	7mg	8mg	4mg	2mg	20mg
Concerta XL 54	54mg	7mg	14mg	13mg	11mg	45mg
Concerta XL 63	63mg	9mg	16mg	16mg	12mg	52.5mg
Equasym XL	30mg	9mg	11mg	6mg	4mg	30mg
Methylphenidate plain	15mg	9mg	6mg	–	–	15mg
Concerta XL 72	72mg	10mg	18mg	18mg	14mg	60mg
Medikinet XL	30mg	10mg	12mg	6mg	3mg	30mg
Equasym XL	40mg	12mg	15mg	8mg	5mg	40mg
Methylphenidate plain	20mg	13mg	7mg	–	–	20mg
Medikinet XL	40mg	13mg	15mg	8mg	3mg	40mg
Equasym XL	50mg	15mg	19mg	10mg	6mg	50mg
Methylphenidate plain	25mg	16mg	9mg	–	–	25mg
Medikinet XL	50mg	17mg	19mg	10mg	4mg	50mg
Equasym XL	60mg	18mg	22mg	12mg	7mg	60mg
Methylphenidate plain	30mg	19mg	11mg	–	–	30mg

Appendix 5a   (Continued)

Product	Stated content	0–4h	4–8h	8–12h	>12h	Total release
Medikinet XL	60mg	20mg	23mg	12mg	5mg	60mg
Equasym XL	70mg	21mg	26mg	14mg	8mg	70mg
Methylphenidate plain	35mg	22mg	13mg	–	–	35mg
Medikinet XL	70mg	23mg	27mg	14mg	6mg	70mg
Equasym XL	80mg	24mg	30mg	16mg	10mg	80mg
Methylphenidate plain	40mg	25mg	15mg	–	–	40mg
Medikinet XL	80mg	27mg	31mg	16mg	7mg	80mg
Equasym XL	90mg	27mg	33mg	18mg	11mg	90mg
Methylphenidate plain	45mg	28mg	17mg	–	–	45mg
Medikinet XL	90mg	30mg	35mg	18mg	8mg	90mg
Methylphenidate plain	50mg	32mg	18mg	–	–	50mg

Courtesy: Reproduced by Professor Steve Bazire

Disclaimers:

1. Chart assumes dose(s) are taken at the correct time (e.g. before, with or after food; slower transit can increase absorption).
2. Confidence intervals are not known so these assume a uniform release.
3. Concerta XL® is reported not to release its full content so the actual release may be around 15% less than the stated content.
4. Calculations are based on proportions of the AUC (Area Under the Curve).
5. It is presumed that Xenidate XL® and Matoride XL® are equivalent to Concerta XL®, although the available data is limited.
6. Different products can be mixed e.g. IR and XL, different XLs, and omitted on some days e.g. weekends.

Thanks to Prof Peter Hill, Dr Val Harpin, Dr Chris Steer, Prof David Coghill and Dr Adrian Brooke for inspiration and for help with this. Reproduced courtesy of Prof. Stephen Bazire, Choice and Medication™ 2016.

Appendix 5b   Comparison of stimulants for the symptoms of ADHD

Non-stimulant medicines are also available e.g. atomoxetine and guanfacine

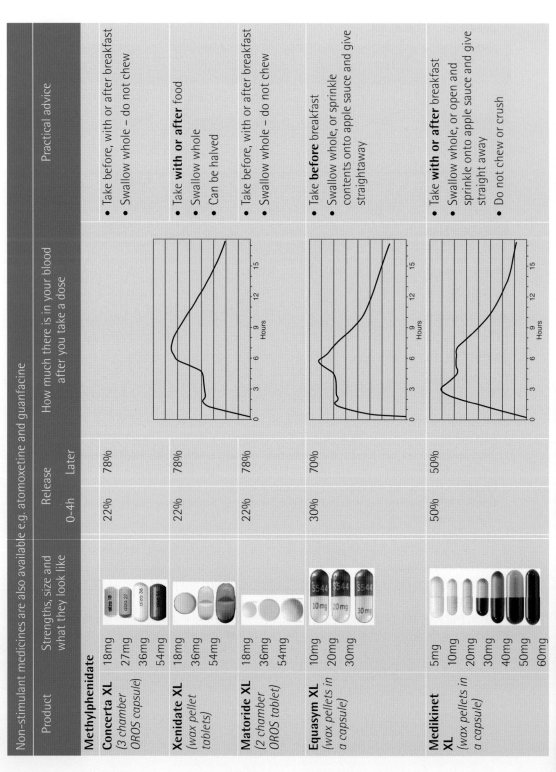

Product	Strengths, size and what they look like	Release 0–4h	Release Later	How much there is in your blood after you take a dose	Practical advice
Methylphenidate					
Concerta XL *(3 chamber OROS capsule)*	18mg 27mg 36mg 54mg	22%	78%		• Take before, with or after breakfast • Swallow whole – do not chew
Xenidate XL *(wax pellet tablets)*	18mg 36mg 54mg	22%	78%		• Take **with or after** food • Swallow whole • Can be halved
Matoride XL *(2 chamber OROS tablet)*	18mg 36mg 54mg	22%	78%		• Take before, with or after breakfast • Swallow whole – do not chew
Equasym XL *(wax pellets in a capsule)*	10mg 20mg 30mg	30%	70%		• Take **before** breakfast • Swallow whole, or sprinkle contents onto apple sauce and give straightaway
Medikinet XL *(wax pellets in a capsule)*	5mg 10mg 20mg 30mg 40mg 50mg 60mg	50%	50%		• Take **with or after** breakfast • Swallow whole, or open and sprinkle onto apple sauce and give straight away • Do not chew or crush

Appendix 5b (Continued)

Non-stimulant medicines are also available e.g. atomoxetine and guanfacine

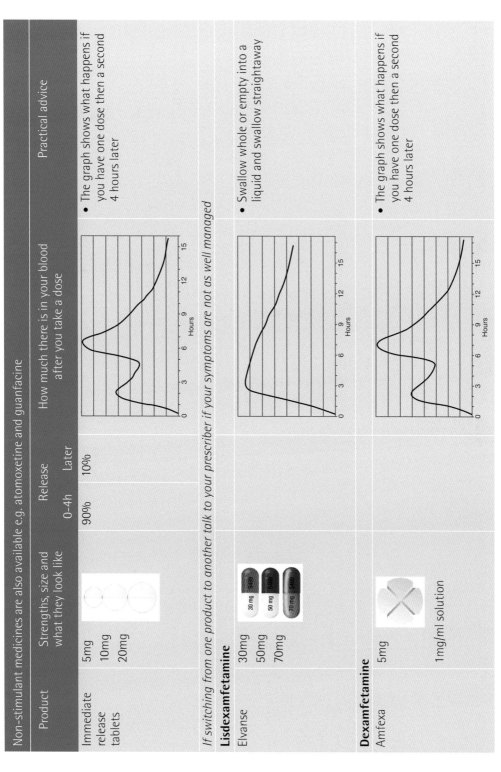

Product	Strengths, size and what they look like	Release 0-4h	Later	How much there is in your blood after you take a dose	Practical advice
Immediate release tablets	5mg 10mg 20mg	90%	10%		• The graph shows what happens if you have one dose then a second 4 hours later

If switching from one product to another talk to your prescriber if your symptoms are not as well managed

Lisdexamfetamine

Elvanse	30mg 50mg 70mg				• Swallow whole or empty into a liquid and swallow straightaway

Dexamfetamine

Amfexa	5mg 1mg/ml solution				• The graph shows what happens if you have one dose then a second 4 hours later

Thanks to Prof Peter Hill, Dr Val Harpin, Dr Chris Steer, Prof David Coghill and Dr Adrian Brooke for inspiration and for help with this. Reproduced courtesy of Prof. Stephen Bazire, Choice and Medication™ 2016.

Index

Recent titles from Mac Keith Press www.mackeith.co.uk

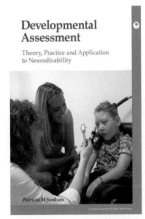

Developmental Assessment: Theory, Practice and Application to Neurodisability
Patricia M. Sonksen

A practical guide from Mac Keith Press
2016 ▪ 384pp ▪ softback ▪ 978-1-909962-56-9
£39.95 / €56.50 / $65.00

This handbook presents a new approach to assessing development in preschool children that can be applied across the developmental spectrum. The reader is taught how to confirm whether development is typical and if it is not, is signposted to the likely nature and severity of impairments, with a plan of action. The author uses numerous case vignettes from her 40 years' experience to bring to life her approach with clear summary key points and helpful illustrations.

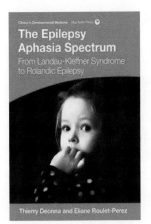

The Epilepsy Aphasia Spectrum: From Landau-Kleffner Syndrome to Rolandic Epilepsy
Thierry Deonna and Elaine Roulet-Perez

Clinics in Developmental Medicine
November 2016 ▪ 200pp ▪ hardback ▪ 978-1-909962-76-7
£50.00 / €62.94 / $75.00

This book starts with a historical look at Landau-Kleffner syndrome (LKS), from the first reported cases to the recognition of the direct role of epileptic activity in language loss or regression, the hallmark of this syndrome. It shows the links between LKS, epilepsy with continuous spike waves during sleep and rolandic epilepsy with its variants that led to the concept of the 'epilepsy-aphasia spectrum'.

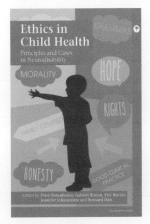

Ethics in Child Health: Principles and Cases in Neurodisability
Peter L. Rosenbaum, Gabriel M. Ronen, Eric Racine, Jennifer Johannesen and Bernard Dan (Editors)

2016 ▪ 396pp ▪ softback ▪ 978-1-909962-63-7
£39.95 / €50.00 / $60.00

This book explores the ethical dimensions of issues that have either been ignored or not recognised. Each chapter is built around an illustrative scenario and discusses how ethical principles can be utilised to inform decision-making. 'Themes for Discussion' at the end of each chapter will help professionals and policy makers put practical ethical thinking at the heart of care.

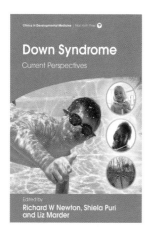

Down Syndrome: Current Perspectives
Richard W. Newton, Shiela Puri and Liz Marder (Editors)

Clinics in Developmental Medicine
2015 ▪ 320pp ▪ hardback ▪ 978-1-909962-47-7
£95.00 / €128.30 / $150.00

Down syndrome remains the most common recognisable form of intellectual disability. The challenge for doctors today is how to capture the rapidly expanding body of scientific knowledge and devise models of care to meet the needs of individuals and their families. *Down Syndrome: Current Perspectives* provides doctors and other health professionals with the information they need to address the challenges that can present in the management of this syndrome.

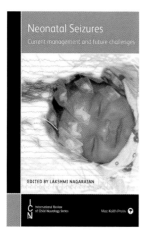

Neonatal Seizures: Current Management and Future Challenges
Lakshmi Nagarajan (Editor)

International Review of Child Neurology Series
2016 ▪ 214pp ▪ hardback ▪ 978-1-909962-67-5
£44.99 / €58.40 / $65.00

This book distils what is known about the many advances in the management of neonatal seizures into one scholarly yet practical text. Chapters cover the neonatal neuron, the use of video EEG in diagnosis, advances in neurophysiology, genetics and neuroprotective strategies, as well as outcomes. This volume will be of use to neonatologists, paediatricians, neurologists and all health professionals involved in the care of neonates experiencing seizures.

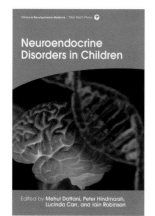

Neuroendocrine Disorders in Children
Mehul Dattani, Peter Hindmarsh, Lucinda Carr and Iain Robinson (Editors)

Clinics in Developmental Medicine
2016 ▪ 424pp ▪ hardback ▪ 978-1-909962-50-7
£74.95 / €105.90 / $120.00

Impairments in the endocrine system can lead to a number of disorders in children including diabetes mellitus, Addison's disease, growth disorders, and Graves' disease among others. This book provides a comprehensive examination of these disorders from infancy to adolescence. This text will be indispensable reading for paediatric endocrinologists, trainee paediatricians, neurologists and adult neurologists.